MW00915911

Certified Orthopaedic Surgery Coder (COSC) Exam Study Guide 2019 Edition

Copyright © Medical Coding Pro
All rights reserved.

ISBN: 9781795831826

DEDICATION

To the hard working students preparing for the certification exam. Your work ethic and dedication to the medical industry will ensure its health and competency for years to come!

Copyright Medical Coding Pro
Published by: IPC Marketing LLC
PO Box 3824
Youngstown, Ohio 44513

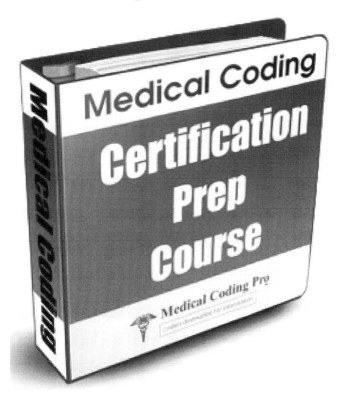

Quick Start Guide

Start by reviewing everything included inside the exam study guide. Contents include the following:

1) Medical Coding Exam Strategy
2) Overview
3) Mock Practice Exam Questions & Answers
4) Secrets To Reducing Exam Stress
5) Common Anatomical Terminology
6) Medical Terminology Prefixes, Roots, and Suffixes
7) Notes
8) Scoring Sheets
9) Resources

These resources will give you a good base to prepare for the board exam.

If you have any questions please email contact us at support@medicalcodingpro.com.

Medical Coding Exam Strategy

One of the first things we should discuss is what "The Strategy" is and what it isn't.

What it is:

A simple, yet powerful, method for increasing your chances of passing the certification exam. Many people have told us that time management was their biggest obstacle in passing the exam. This is what "The Strategy" addresses. It is a road map to pass the exam. It has very little to do with coding knowledge and everything to do with your approach.

What it isn't:

A long, drawn out, hard to follow maze with do's and don'ts reviewing the material that was covered in class. We assume that you know the material, otherwise, it doesn't matter what we teach you the odds are against you.

Why it is important: The reality is many people do not pass the exam the first time. This becomes a costly proposition and one that wasn't bargained for because the next step is an exam retake. The cost: $380. Some even go further and sign up for a three day "boot camp". The cost: about $1200.

Between a rock and a hard place

In this very typical example you passed the Medical Coding class with flying colors but the major hospitals and doctor offices all want a certified medical coder. Why, because it increases their output, makes them more money, and limits their liability for mistakes. So now you're stuck. You have to get certified, but at what cost? It all depends how many times you have to take the certification exam. Follow the steps outlined in "The Strategy" and your next exam could reward you with a certification.

Start by reviewing common mistakes

Some of the most common mistakes made while taking the exam are what we like to call "time wasters". The most important factor to succeeding is time management. You only have 5 hours and 40 minutes to complete the exam (including breaks) and it consists of 150 questions so every minute counts.

The time breakdown goes like this: Exam Time (without breaks) 5 hours 40 minutes or 340 minutes. Exam length: 150 Questions. The easy math is two minute per question. What can we eliminate to save time?

Things Not To Do

1) Answer each question in numerical order.
2) Take too much time on difficult questions first.
3) Read the doctors chart before reading the detail of the question.
4) Not highlighting questions "passed" in the first round

Time Waster #1:

Answering each question in numerical order

If you answer each question in numerical order you will never finish the exam! This is one of the most common mistakes made. If you start out answering the first several questions just fine and then ten questions into the exam you come to a one that you have trouble with, what then? This is a "time burner" and one you can not get hung up on. We will review why this is more important later in "The Strategy".

The Exam is five hours and forty minutes and 150 questions... an average of two minutes per question. The key is to redistribute your time.

Time Waster #2:

Taking too much time on difficult questions the first time through the exam

"The Strategy" is based on a "two pass" system. The first pass is designed to answer the easy questions and highlight the more difficult ones. These will be addressed on the second pass. A good rule of thumb is if you can't answer it in a minute and a half, move on! If you continue to work on these questions you run the risk of not completing the exam or having to rush through the more difficult questions at the end.

Time Waster #3:

Reading the doctors chart before reading the detail of the question

If you get caught in this "time waster" it will rob you of valuable minutes. Always read the question completely before reading the doctors chart. You may be able to eliminate much of the chart because the question is requesting limited information or specific detail.

Time waster #4:

Not highlighting the more difficult questions for the second "pass"

Be prepared. Have a game plan and stick to it. Make sure that you highlight the more difficult questions that you are going to "pass" on in the first round of the exam. If you make the mistake of not highlighting these questions, you will lose valuable minutes trying to search for them in the second round.

Your goal is to answer the easier questions in a minute and a half maximum! Out of 150 questions, let's assume you can answer 60%, or 90 questions, on the first pass averaging 1 minutes per question. That is a total of 135 minutes to answer the first 90 questions. Again, this is an average. That leaves you with 165 minutes to answer the remaining 60 questions. That comes out to 2 minutes per question on the second pass! Now you can be more deliberate with the remaining, more difficult, questions to make sure you answer them correctly.

The "time wasters" have to be minimized or eliminated for you to be successful. Every minute you can save on looking up codes or moving more difficult questions to the second pass the closer you are to your certification.

"Time Wasters" have to be avoided at all costs. Implement a "two pass" system and watch your results increase substantially!

Now let's take an in depth look at the keys that will make all the difference in your exam experience. These are "The Strategy" and "The "Keys" to passing a certification exam! These are not difficult, complex strategies. These are straight forward, simple strategies that are easy to implement and highly effective. Follow each step and you will be well on your way to certification.

The Exam Strategy:

1) The basic element of the strategy is making two passes through the exam. The first pass is to answer the questions you can complete in 1 . minute or less. This should be about 60% of the questions. If you can not answer a question in that time, highlight it (mark it for the second pass) and move on! That creates 2 minutes for the remaining 40% which you have identified as more difficult. This should leave you plenty of time on the more difficult questions and improve your overall score.

2) Answer the easier questions in each section on the first pass. You have to answer 70% of the questions or better correctly to pass so answering the easier questions in each section will form a good base of correctly answered questions in all sections thus improving your chances of passing.

3) Identify the first three numbers of the code first. This will help you eliminate answers instantly and narrow your choices for the correct answer. This is a big "time saver". Practice this on your mock practice exam.

4) Read each question before reading the entire doctors chart. Another big "time saver"! Don't waste valuable time reading the entire doctors chart before reading the question. Read the entire question first to find out the specific information the question is requesting.

5) Highlight Procedures one color, Diagnosis another color and Modifiers a third color for quick reference (again, a big time saver!)

The Keys to Success:

Key #1: Study and Preparation.

Don't let anyone fool you into thinking that you don't have to study. That is not the case. You NEED to study, and study hard! The Exam Strategy assumes that you know all the material. There are no shortcuts and The Exam Strategy will only help you pass if you know the material. So put in the time!

One of the best tools available to practice time management for the exam is the Medical Coding Exam System

(www.MedicalCodingExamSystem.com).

It is course dedicated strictly to time management. This will pay big dividends during the exam. We also highly the Faster Coder (www.fastercoder.com) to improve your speed and accuracy. You will quickly find it is worth its weight in gold.

Key #2: Two Complete Passes through the Exam.

During the exam you will be making TWO passes through the entire exam. Let me repeat this because it is at the heart of what we are trying to accomplish. During the exam you will be going through the entire exam twice! The first pass is to answer the easier questions and the second pass is to answer the more difficult ones. Many people do not pass the exam because they get caught up on a few difficult questions and end up not completing the entire exam. You must follow this key element as it is your key to success.

Key #3: Answer The First Pass Questions in 1 1/2 Minutes or Less.

Start the exam by making a first pass. During the first pass answer all the questions that you can complete in a reasonable amount of time (1 1/2 minutes). If you can't answer the question in 1 1/2 minutes highlight it and move on!

Key #4: Highlight All Unanswered Questions in First Pass

If you cannot answer a question within 1 1/2 minutes of the first pass, highlight the unanswered questions in yellow for easy reference during the second pass! Do not forget to highlight them as every second counts and this could be a big time saver!

Key #5: Answer the More Difficult Questions during Second Pass

You should complete the first pass in 135 minutes or less. This will establish a good base of answered questions and leave you with 165 minutes or more to go back and answer the highlighted questions.

Key #6: Do Not Answer the Questions in Order, You Will Fail!

If you take your time and answer the first 80% of questions perfect but run out of time and have to guess on the remaining 20% questions, YOU WILL NOT PASS. You must answer 70% of the questions correctly to pass the exam!

Key #7: Identify the First Three Numbers of the Code

Another good "time saver" is to identify the first three numbers of the code, turn to that page, then go to the sub code numbers.

Key #8: You Can Miss a Certain Percentage in each Section

You can miss a certain percentage in each section and still pass the exam. Your goal is to get enough right to pass. Making two complete passes through the exam will ensures that you are, at minimum, answering the easy questions in each section first. This alone will increase your chances of passing because you will have a base of questions answered in each section. Typically, the last section is rushed through. This will eliminate this hurdle.

Key #9: Read Each Question before Reading the Doctors Chart

Go over each question before you read the doctors chart. This will tell you exactly what you are looking for. You may not need to read the entire chart because the question only references a specific section. This will save you precious time.

Key #10: Highlight Procedures, Diagnosis, and Modifiers

Highlight the patient's treatment/s in different colors for easy reference. I recommend using these colors: Yellow for Procedures, Blue for Diagnosis, and Pink for Modifiers.

Key #11: You Must Answer 70% correctly to pass the exam

You must keep moving! Leave the tough questions and move on. Ask around to anyone who did not pass the exam the first time (or more) and see what they say. It's all about time management and using the right tips and techniques. So to that end, if you do not follow any other advice, follow this! Do the easiest questions first.

Bonus Tips:

1) Eliminate any answers that begin with an V-Code instantly! Cross it out... this will reduce your selection of answers.

2) Code injections with an administration charge.

3) Supervision and Interpretation components require physician supervision. In radiology procedures this means the radiologist has participated.

4) Know the difference between modifier 26 and modifier TC from your HCPCS II book.

5) Diabetes mellitus – etiology code first then the manifestation code.

6) Trauma accident- always code the most severe injury first

7) Tab all your books including CPT, HCPCS Level II, ICD-10-CM, for quick reference.

8) Code burns on the depth of the burn (1st, 2nd, or 3rd degree). Burns are classified to the extent of the body surface involved. When coding burns of multiple sites, assign separate codes for each burn site. Also burns of the same local site (three-character category level, T20-T28), but of different degrees should be coded to the highest degree documented.

9) Multiple fractures, code by site and sequence by severity.

10) If the same bone is fractured or dislocated, code the fracture only.

11) If the question doesn't state open or closed fracture, code as a closed fracture.

12) Late effects (now called "sequela); is a residual of previous illness or injury. Code the residual and then the cause. Reference "late" in the index.

13) Sequence symptoms first if no diagnosis.

14) Study Medicare A, B, C, D

15) Understand modifier 62 co-surgeons (look on exam for surgeon A and B)

16) ***KEEP MOVING, KEEP MOVING, AND KEEP MOVING!***

Overview

Certified Orthopaedic Surgery Coder (COSC)

The Certified Orthopaedic Surgery Coder (COSC™) exam was developed by a team of leading orthopaedic coding professionals. Coders with sufficient experience and expertise in orthopaedic coding are encouraged to sit for the COSC™ exam.

COSC examinees will be tested on:

- Ability to read and abstract physician office notes and procedure notes to apply correct ICD-10-CM, CPT®, HCPCS Level II and modifier coding assignments
- Evaluation and management (both the 1995 and 1997 Documentation Guidelines)
- Rules and regulations of Medicare billing including (but not limited to) incident to, teaching situations, shared visits, consultations and global surgery
- Coding of surgical procedures performed by orthopedists such as arthroscopic surgeries, fracture repairs, spine surgeries, etc.
- Medical terminology
- Anatomy and physiology

The COSC Exam

- 150 multiple choice questions (proctored)

- 5 hours and 40 minutes to finish the exam

- One free retake

- $350

- Open code book (manuals)

Mock Practice Exam Questions & Answers

The following is a Medical Coding Pro mock practice exam. You may not use any outside materials for this exam other than the manuals referenced by the American Academy of Professional Coders (AAPC ©).

The code research program we use and recommend is Find A Code. You can locate it at: www.findacode.com?pc=MEDCOPRO.

To pass the certification exam you must manage your time carefully. If after going through this practice you determine that time management is a skill you may need additional assistance with, the Medical Coding Exam System (www.MedicalCodingExamSystem.com) is an excellent resource for additional support.

If you want additional resources to prepare for the certification exam we highly recommend FasterCoder.com (www.FasterCoder.com).

COSC Mock Exam - 100 Questions

20,000 Series (musculoskeletal)

1. Bob, a construction worker, has pain in his hand and fingers from operating a caulk gun. It requires decompression. Code the procedure (injection injury):

a. 26010
b. 26035
c. 26105
d. 25927

2. Codes 21076 to 21089 should be used for:

a. Prosthesis prepared by an outside lab
b. Prosthesis of the lower leg and foot.
c. Prosthesis of the lower arm and hand.
d. Prosthesis actually designed and prepared by the physician.

3. To bill for the diagnostic arthroscopy with a surgical arthroscopy:

a. Code 29800 to 29847 plus the appropriate surgical procedure.
b. Diagnostic arthroscopy is included with surgical arthroscopy. Don't bill it
c. Add Modifier -61.
d. Code 29800, 29999 and the surgical procedure.

4. What code is used to describe using heat to shrink a capsule in the shoulder via arthroscopic procedure?

a. 17000
b. 17313
c. 46917
d. No specific code use 29999 - unlisted procedure.

5. Arthrodesis means:

a. Attaching a ligament to a bone
b. Fusing bones together
c. Connecting two veins or arteries together.
d. Using a catheter to expand an occluded vessel.

6. Spinal Instrumentation means:

a. Fixation at each end of the construct and at least one additional
   interposed bony attachment.
b. Instruments that are used to diagnose, analyze and report imperfections
   in the back.
c. A back brace that is worn at night.
d. Instruments used to test the nerve impulse of the spinal cord.

7. Using an anterior approach, the physician fused C5 and C6. Code for this
procedure.

a. 22554
b. 22556
c. 22558
d. 22558-50

8. Report the exploration of spinal fusion:

a. 22830
b. 22830-26
c. 22830-32
d. 22830-52

9. A methylmethacrylate replacement was applied to correct a vertebral defect.

a. 22845
b. 22853
c. 22840
d. 22842

10. Instrumentation procedures (22840 - 22855):

a. Include the surgical procedure, no modifier necessary
b. Report in addition to codes for the procedures with modifier -22
c. Report in addition to codes for the procedures without modifier -51
d. Report in addition to codes for the procedures with modifier -51

11. Code for a closed reduction and percutaneous pin fixation of fracture, left middle finger.

a. 26755
b. 26755-F2
c. 26756-F2
d. 26755-F2, 26756-F2

12. Code for closed reduction of radial shaft fracture; With manipulation.

a. 25505-22
b. 25505
c. 25505-52
d. 25535

13. The physician performed a transverse incision of the tendon at the base of the patient's thumb to release the contracture:

a. 26502
b. 26390
c. 26508
d. 26510

14. Laminectomy is:

a. Destruction via laser of the vertebral lamina.
b. Excision of a vertebral lamina; commonly used to denote removal of the posterior arch.
c. Incision between the vertabral lamina and the septum pellucidem.
d. Excision of the Laminoleous Molluscom.

15. Code for a partial medial arthroscopic meniscectomy of the knee with limited debridement.

a. 21060
b. 29880
c. 29881
d. 29881, 29897

16. Mary, a 40 year old executive secretary has developed marked pain along her radioscaphoid and radiolunate joints. After a radiograph fails to reveal the problem, she is scheduled for diagnostic arthroscopy under local anesthesia. Code for both procedures:

a. 29830, 01829
b. 29840, 01829
c. 29840, 01829-23
d. None of the answers are correct.

17. A decompression fasciotomy is:

a. An excision of all or part of the fascia, due to necrosis.
b. An incision through the fascia to relieve pressure, where an injury or disorder could interrupt blood flow.
c. The placement of a stent into the fascia to relieve pressure, where an injury or disorder could interrupt blood flow.
d. The repair or fixation of the facial ligaments, where an injury or disorder could interrupt blood flow.

18. Transtemporal approach

a. Above the temple.
b. Below the temple.
c. Common approach for a frontal lobotomy.
d. None of the Answers are correct.

19. Disarticulation (at knee)

a. A severe sprain, but no bones are broken.
b. A severe break of the bones.
c. Amputation of limb through the joint, without cutting of the bone.
d. A degenerative disease of the cartilage.

20. Bone grafting

a. Bone fragments or bone pegs are used for transplant in the area of the lesion.
b. Shaping or scraping of a bone to remove a prominence.
c. Excising bone fragments or cartilage from a cavity or spaces (such as the knee).
d. None of the above are correct.

21. The physician's Operative Report stated, "ablation of three osteoid osteomas via RFA, with CT Guidance." Code for the procedure(s).

a. 20982
b. 20982 X 3
c. 20982 X 3, 77014
d. 20982, 20999 X 2, 77014

22. The surgeon performed arthrodesis of the vertebral bodies, L1, L2 and L3 (total of 3), using a lateral extracavitoary approach of L1 (lumbar). A minimal diskectomy was performed to prepare the interspace.

a. 22533
b. 22533-22
c. 22533 X 3
d. 22533 + 22534 X 2

23. Code for a musculoskeletal functional capacity test, 30 minutes. with report.

a. 97750
b. 97750-26
c. 97750 X 2
d. 97750-26 X 2

24. Code 22556, arthrodesis is often performed:

a. In an ambulatory Surgery Center..
b. By two physicians.
c. Under local Anesthesia.
d. By a NeuroSurgeon.

25. An allograft would most likely be obtained from:

a. Patient
b. Patient's relative
c. Anyone with the same tissue type.
d. A cadaver

26. Closed treatment means that a bone is broken and:

a. There is no open wound in the skin and the fracture site does not have to be surgically opened to be repaired.
b. Treatment is performed in a "closed" or sterile room environment.
c. That treatment of the fracture is all performed laparoscopically.
d. None of the answers are correct.

27. A joint aspiration,

a. or arthrocentesis,
b. is a procedure whereby a sterile needle and syringe are used to drain fluid from the joint.
c. Both answers are correct.
d. None of the answers are correct.

28. The rotator cuff is:

a. A group of circular tendons that fuse together and surround the front of the shoulder joint like a cuff on a shirt sleeve.

b. A group of long tendons that fuse together and surround the front and back of the shoulder joint like a cuff on a shirt sleeve.

c. A group of short tendons that fuse together and surround the top and bottom of the shoulder joint like a cuff on a shirt sleeve.

d. A group of flat tendons that fuse together and surround the front, back, and top of the shoulder joint like a cuff on a shirt sleeve.

29. What codes are used to report a repair of a rotator cuff?

a. 23400 to 24341 and 29827
b. 23410 to 24341
c. 23410 to 24341 and 29827
d. 23410 to 24346 and 29827

30. Meniscal tears are divided into

a. Traumatic and non-traumatic tears
b. Distal and Proximal tears
c. Anterior and Posterior tears
d. Basic and Complex tears

31. Code for an open I & D of a lumbosacral deep abscess.

a. 22010
b. 22015
c. 22010, 22850
d. 22015, 22850

32. A meniscectomy refers to:

a. Arthrotomy and arthroscopy codes of the knee.
b. Excision of a meniscus from the knee joint.
c. Excision of a meniscus from the the temporomandibular joint.
d. All of the answers are correct.

33. Code for bilateral Percutaneous Vertebroplasty with fluoroscopic guidance.

a. 22510
b. 22510-RT; 22510-LT
c. 22510-50
d. None of the answers are correct

34. What types of guidance are used for Percutaneous Vertebroplasty (answer is in the Cigna Policy Statement)

a. Fluoroscopic and/or CT guidance
b. X-Ray only
c. MRI or CT
d. CT, X-Ray, Spect and Fluoroscopy

35. What is the most common approach for total disc arthroplasty?

a. Posterior
b. Lateral
c. Transverse
d. Anterior

36. The physician performed a transverse incision of the tendon at the base of the patient's thumb to release the contracture.

a. 26502
b. 26390
c. 26508
d. 26510

37. Which code is used to describe using heat to shrink a capsule in the shoulder via arthroscopic procedure? DUPLICATE

a. 23040
b. 29805
c. 29806
d. Use 29999 - unlisted procedure.

38. Code for a Total disc arthroplasty (artificial disc), anterior approach, including discectomy w/ end plate prep (incl ostephytectomy for nerve root or spinal cord decompression and microdissection), single interspace, cervical

a. 22856
b. 22861
c. 22862
d. 0098T.

39. How do you code for the removal of a 10 cm. Lipoma from the soft tissue of the shoulder of a 55 year old mailman?

a. 23071
b. 23073
c. 23075 X 2
d. 23075

40. Code for radical resection of a tumor of the clavicle.

a. 23200
b. 23210
c. 23220
d. 23330

41. Code for the radical resection of a 2 cm malignant tumor from the soft tissue of the right

a. 24077-RT
b. 24077
c. 24079-50
d. 24079-RT

42. Code for the removal of a 3 cm tumor from the soft tissue of the left forearm.

a. 25071
b. 25071-LT
c. 25075
d. 25075-LT

43. Code for the removal of a 2 cm vascular malformation of the soft tissue of the left thumb.

a. 26111-FA
b. 26111-LT
c. 26113-FA
d. 26113-LT

44. Code for the removal of a subcutaneous 3 cm tumor from the soft tissue of the right hip.

a. 27043
b. 27043-RT
c. 27047
d. 27047-RT

45. Code for the excision of a 6 cm subcutaneous tumor from the soft tissue of the right leg.

a. 27632
b. 27632-RT
c. 27632 X 2
d. 27632-50

46. Code for the excision of a 1cm intramuscular tumor from the soft tissue of the left foot, third digit.

a. 28041-T2
b. 28041-T3
c. 28045-T2
d. 28045-T3

47. The physician first applied strapping then, shortly after, multiple layers of a venous wound compression just below the patient's left knee.

a. 29581
b. 29581-LT, 29540
c. 29581-LT
d. 29581X2

Medical Terminology

48. Intramuscular means:

a. Within the substance of the skin
b. Within a corpuscle
c. Beneath the skin
d. Within the substance of the muscle

49. Excessive concavity in the lumbar region of the spine:

a. Scoliosis
b. Kyphosis
c. Lordosis
d. Mentosis

50. Excessive convexity in the thoracic region of the spine:

a. Scoliosis
b. Kyphosis
c. Lordosis
d. Mentosis

51. Lateral curvature of the spine:

a. Scoliosis
b. Kyphosis
c. Lordosis
d. Mentosis

52. Superficial fascia is:

a. Just above the subcutaneous tissue
b. Just under the subcutaneous tissue
c. Beneath the first layer of muscle
d. Just below the dermis

53. Arthroplasty means

a. The insertion of a plastic stent into an artery
b. It is an arthritic condition of the bones
c. Repair of cartilage
d. Joint repair

54. A laminectomy is:

a. Destruction via laser of the vertebral lamina.
b. Excision of a vertebral lamina; commonly used to denote removal of the
       posterior arch.
c. Incision between the vertabral lamina and the septum pellucidem.
d. Excision of the Laminoleous Molluscom.

55. Osteo - myelitis

a. Neoplasm in bone that results in thinning and fragmentation
b. Inflammation of the bone marrow and adjacent bone.
c. Excessive formation of dense trabecular bone and calcified cartilage
d. A bony outgrowth or protuberance.

56. Arthrodesis means:

a. Attaching a ligament to a bone
b. Fusing bones together
c. Inserting a stent through a cannula into a fistula
d. Reattaching muscle to a tendon

57. Osteo - penia

a. Hardening of the penis.
b. Decreased calcification of the bone
c. Shrinking of the bone.
d. Inflammation of the bone marrow.

58. Osteo - periostitis

a. Inflammation of the bone marrow.
b. Morbid process in bone (condition)
c. Benign mass in the bone.
d. Malignant mass in the bone.

59. Osteo - petrosis

a. Mottled or spotted bones
b. Porous condition of the bones.
c. Excessive formation of dense trabecular bone and calcified cartilage
d. Neoplasm in bone that results in thinning and fragmentation

60. Osteo - phyte

a. Benign mass
b. Malignant mass
c. Inflammation of the bone.
d. A bony outgrowth or protuberance.

61. Osteo - plasty

a. Grafting, reparative or plastic surgery of bones.
b. Cutting of a bone
c. Internal fixation of a fracture, common by screw, pin or plate.
d. Suture - wiring together fragments of broken bone.

62. Osteopoikilosis means:

a. Mottled or spotted bones.
b. Reduced calcification of bones.
c. Deterioration of bone mass.
d. Removing bone marrow from the bone.

63. Osteo - porosis

a. Porous condition of bone.
b. Atrophy of skeletal tissue.
c. Swelling of bone.
d. Hardening of the bone.

64. Osteo - porotic

a. Deterioration of the bone.
b. Porous condition of the bones.
c. Nutrition of osseous tissue.
d. Abnormal hardening of bones.

65. Osteo - radionecrosis means:

a. Healing of the bone via an electrical current.
b. Magnetic Resonance Imaging of the bone. (MRI)
c. Reduced calcification of the bone.
d. Deterioration of bone produced by ionizing radiation.

66. Osteo - rrhaphy means:

a. Disease of the bone
b. Destruction of the bone
c. Calcification of the bone
d. Wiring together fragments of broken bone (suturing)

67. Osteo - sclerosis

a. Abnormal softening of the bone.
b. Calcification of the bone.
c. Abnormal hardening of bone.
d. Malignancy of the bone

68. Osteo - spongioma

a. Malignant neoplasm of the bone.
b. Calcification of the bone.
c. One or more veins of the bone.
d. Neoplasm in bone that results in thinning and fragmentation.

69. Osteosteatoma means:

a. Malignant mass on the bone.
b. Benign mass of the bone.
c. Atrophy of skeletal tissue.
d. Morbid process of the bone

70. Osteo - thrombosis

a. Calcification of the bone
b. Swelling of the bone.
c. Deterioration of the bone.
d. Clotting within one or more veins of the bone.

71. Osteo - tribe

a. Disease of the bone marrow.
b. Fragments of bone
c. Instrument for analysis of bone.
d. Instrument for crushing off bits of bone.

72. From the wrist the order of the bones of the hand are:

a. Carpal bones, metacarpal bones and phalanges.
b. Metacarpal bones, Carpal bones and phalanges.
c. Tarsal bones, metatarsal bones and phalanges.
d. Carpal bones, metatarsal bones and phalanges.

73. The parietal bone is:

a. At the base of the skull,
b. The largest bone of the skull, superior to the occipital bone.
c. Anterior to the Frontal bone and Posterior to the occipital bone.
d. The bone on the side of the skull where the ear is.

74. The number of ribs is _____ and they correspond to _____ of the spinal column.

a. 8, L1 - L8
b. 12, T1 - T 12
c. 12, T1 - S5
d. 24, T1 - S4

75. Osteo - trophy

a. Nutrition of osseous tissue.
b. Deterioration of bone tissue.
c. Calcification of bone tissue.
d. Swelling of bone tissue

76. Laminectomy

a. Lamination of a cortisal layer around the arachnoid foramen
b. The lamina are large, thick nerves intertwined between vertabrae C1, C2 and T1. This is an excision of the excess, hardened growth.
c. An incision into the plate or layer of the vertabrae.
d. Surgical excision of the lamina of the vertebra.

77. Replantation

a. The surgical reconstruction of a body part from another. (.i.e., using cartilage from another site to reconstruct and ear)
b. The replacement (reattachment) of an organ to its original site.
c. Setting a bone back into its original position.
d. Increasing the number of red blood cells in the medulla ossium.

78. Epiphyseal arrest

a. Fixation of a compound fracture with pins and screws.
b. Bone lengthening or shortening.
c. A rare condition where the bones no longer grow. Their growth is essentially "arrested."
d. A graft of the epiphyseal bone to strengthen it after a fracture.

79. Laminotomy

a. An incision into the lamina.
b. Removal of the intervertebral foramen.
c. A complete removal of the vertebral lamina.
d. A partial removal of the vertebral lamina.

80. Osteotomy

a. A degenerative disease of the bones.
b. Removal of a small piece or sliver of bone for grafting.
c. Creating a small incision into a bone to aspirate bone marrow.
d. Using a saw to cut the bone.

81. Percutaneous skeletal fixation means:

a. The fracture fragments are visualized and fixation (such as pins) is placed across the fracture site.
b. In this procedure, the fracture fragments are not visualized, but fixation (such as pins) is placed across the fracture site, usually under x-ray imaging.
c. This is considered a closed treatment.
d. None of the above are correct.

82. Arthrodesis

a. Creation of a juncture between to vessels or body parts.
b. A degenerative disease of the cartilage.
c. Fusing bones together.
d. A degenerative disease of the bone.

83. Open Treatment:

a. Refers to a fracture site not surgically opened but no cast is applied, therefore the treatment is considered "open."
b. To fixing a fracture with a "soft" or flexible cast.
c. Is when the core of the bone is hollowed out and new bone marrow is transplanted (bone marrow transplant).
d. Is when a fracture is surgically opened and exposed to the external environment.

84. C1-C2

a. Includes the primos and hexis vertabra
b. The first two cervical vertebra, located in the neck.
c. The first two columnar vertebra, located in the middle of the back.
d. The first two celiac vertebra, located near the sacrum.

85. Osteo - thrombosis

a. Calcification of the bone
b. Swelling of the bone.
c. Deterioration of the bone.
d. Thrombus or clotting within one or more veins of the bone.

86. With manipulation means:

a. Attaching pins, wires and screws to the bone.
b. Using electrical stimulation to promote healing of the fracture.
c. Attaching a cast to the fracture.
d. None of the answers are correct.

87. Traction is:

a. The application of a pushing force to hold a bone in alignment.
b. The application of electricity to aid in the healing of a bone fracture.
c. Using pins, screws and an external fixation device to aid in the healing of a fracture.
d. The application of a pulling force to hold a bone in alignment.

88. A comminuted fracture is

a. Also known as a "hairline" fracture.
b. Broken into several pieces.
c. Repaired fracture.
d. One that does not heal.

89. Vertebroplasty is an

a. Image-guided, minimally invasive, nonsurgical therapy used to strengthen
   a broken spinal bone.
b. Procedure used to treat bones weakened by osteoporosis.
c. Procedure used to treat bones weakened by osteoporosis or cancer.
d. All the answers are correct.

90. When a wound repair requires that blood vessels, tendons, or nerves be
repaired:

a. Report using integumentary codes plus modifier-22 indicating it is a more
   complex procedure than usual.
b. Report using integumentary system codes and the the appropriate body
   system (cardiovascular, musculoskeletal, or nervous).
c. Report using codes from the appropriate body system (cardiovascular,
   musculoskeletal, or nervous).
d. None of the answers are correct.

90,000 Series (medicine)

91. Osteopathic manipulation is found:

a. In the Medicine section of the CPT manual.
b. In the 20000 section, Musculoskeletal.
c. Appendix G.
d. It is not found in the CPT manual at all, because services are not performed by a medical doctor.

92. Codes in the Musculoskeletal section stating "requiring anesthesia" refer to:

a. Any anesthesia
b. Regional and general
c. Conscious sedation
d. General only

93. Code for the exploration and debridement of a wound of a patient shot in the hand during an argument in a bar.

a. 20100
b. 20101
c. 20102
d. 20103

94. Concerning fracture care, "with manipulation" means:

a. Refers to the electrical stimulation of fractured bone to hasten recovery.
b. Reduced, or set (reduction of the fracture)
c. Only refers to extraordinary means and should always include a -22 modifier
d. Interpolation of a fracture.

95. A patient has his hand replanted. This means:

a. A hand was reattached through microsurgery
b. A hand was amputated
c. Skin (autogenous) was grafted onto his hand
d. There is no such term (replanted)

Anatomy

96. Chondromalacia patella is:

a. A common disease of old age.
b. A common disease of young and healthy athletes.
c. A common disease of the ankle.
d. A rare disease of the knee.

97. Dystonia is:

a. A syndrome of gradual muscle atrophy usually producing twisting and repetitive movements or abnormal postures.
b. A syndrome of sustained muscle contractions, usually producing twisting and repetitive movements or abnormal postures.
c. Difficulty of calcium production.
d. Difficulty of walking.

98. A laminotomy is:

a. An excision of the intervertebral discs.
b. An excision of the intervertebral foramen.
c. An excision of a portion of a vertebral lamina.
d. An excision of the entire vertebral lamina.

99. Which vertebrae are fused together?

a. Cervical
b. Thoracic
c. Lumbar
d. Sacral.

100. Code for a chondrocyte implantation, knee. The implantation was a graft from the patient.

a. 27412
b. 27415
c. 27416
d. 27418

COSC Mock Exam - Answers

20,000 Series (musculoskeletal)

1. b. 26035, is an injection injury, caulk gun is essentially the same as a "grease gun" in the CPT example above.

2. d. Prosthesis actually designed and prepared by the physician. This is taken directly from the Guidelines (toward the end) directly proceeding codes 21076 - 21089.

3. b. Diagnostic arthroscopy is included with surgical arthroscopy, Yes, INCLUDED, always, and this is a general rule for all diagnostic / surgical "-scopy" procedures. If you got this question wrong, be sure to read the guidelines proceeding each.

4. d. No specific code; Use Unlisted Code 29999. If a surgical procedure does not match the CPT code, then DON'T code what is closest. Code an UNLISTED procedure and then you will need to send the Operative Report with the Claim Form to get reimbursed. Many unlisted codes are listed in the CPT Assistant Archives or CPT Companion booklet available from the AMA.

5. b. Fusing bones together.

6. a. Fixation at each end of the construct and at least one additional interposed bony attachment is correct.

7. a. 22554 Cervical vertebrae are C1 - C8 Arthrodesis, anterior interbody technique… cervical fusion... below C2.

8. a. 22830 - Exploration of spinal fusion. No modifier is necessary.

9. b. 22853 - application of intervertebral biomechanical devices,

methylmethacrylate, to vertebral defect...

10. c. Instrumentation procedures (22840 - 22855): Report in addition to codes for the procedures without modifier -51, this is the correct and BEST answer. This is directly from the Spinal Instrumentation Guidelines.

11. d. In this scenario you will code for both the closed reduction AND the pin fixation. 26755-F2 - Closed Reduction. 26756-F2 - Percutaneous skeletal fixation of distal phalangeal fracture, finger or thumb, each. F2 is Left Hand - third digit. Skeletal Fixation and External Fixation/Fixator, Percutaneous; External fixation utilizes multiple pins placed through one cortex or both cortices of bone above and below a fracture. These pins are held by an external device, which is called an external fixator. This external fixator is used as an alternative to pins and plaster; it holds the bone fragments in proper position. Pins and plaster also continue to be used in certain clinical situations.

12. b. 25505 - Closed treatment of radial shaft fracture; with manipulation.

13. c. 26508 - release of thenar muscles (e.g., thumb contracture.)

14. b. Laminectomy is the removal of all of the bony arch of a lamina.

15. c. 29881. Arthroscopy, knee, surgical; with meniscectomy (medial *OR* lateral, including any meniscal shaving). The debridement would be included with the meniscectomy code.

16. d. Anesthesia codes are for general anesthesia. Local anesthesia is NOT coded separately.

17. b. Decompression fasciotomy: An incision through the fascia to relieve pressure, where an injury or disorder could interrupt blood flow.

18. d. Transtemporal Approach: Trans: Across ; Temporal: The temple.

19. c. Disarticulation [at knee]: Amputation of limb through the joint, without cutting of the bone.

20. a. Bone Grafting Bone fragments or bone pegs may be obtained from the hip bone (ilium), or an allograft may be used for transplant in the area of the lesion. If the drilling is performed with bone grafting, code 29885 is reported.

21. a. 20982 -Ablation of bone tumor(s) via Radiofrequency Tissue Ablation (RFA). This code includes the CT guidance. Use the one code for one or more tumors. 2007 CPT code 77014 is for the CT guidance for placement of the radiation therapy

22. d. 22532- thoracic, 22533 lumbar 22534 Add-On for either; Answer is 22533 + 22534 X 2 for three bodies. This is a difficult Question.

23. c. 97750 is for a musculoskeletal functional capacity test, per 15 minutes (therefore X 2). WITH REPORT, therefore MOD-26 is redundant and not needed.

24. b. By two physician is the best answer. To code, add MOD-62 to the procedure code for both physicians. Source: AMA CPT Assistant. This would probably be performed in the hospital under full anesthesia by an orthopedic surgeon.

25. d. A cadaver is the best answer.

26. a. Closed treatment means that a bone is broken but there is no open wound in the skin and the fracture site does not have to be surgically opened to be repaired, that is, exposed to the external environment and directly visualized. Laparoscopic is through the abdomen and not likely.

27. c. A joint aspiration, or arthrocentesis, is a procedure whereby a sterile needle and syringe are used to drain fluid from the joint. Joint aspiration is typically performed as an office procedure or at the bedside of hospitalized patients. The purpose of joint aspiration is to obtain joint fluid for examination in the laboratory. Analysis of joint fluid can help to define causes of joint swelling or arthritis, such as infection, gout, and rheumatoid disease. Joint fluid can be tested for white cell count, crystals, protein, glucose, as well as cultured for infection.

28. d. The rotator cuff is a group of flat tendons that fuse together and surround the front, back, and top of the shoulder joint like a cuff on a shirt sleeve.

29. c. The rotator cuff repair codes are 23410 to 24341 and 29827.

30. a. Meniscal tears are divided into traumatic and non-traumatic tears. Traumatic tears can occur in knees that are essentially stable or unstable. Non-traumatic lesions are divided into degenerative and tears seen in conjunction with arthritis.

31. b. 22015 Incision and drainage, open of deep abscess (subfascila), ; lumbar, sacral or lumbosacral.

32. d. All of the answers are correct. Codes 27332, 27333, 29880, and 29881, Arthrotomy and arthroscopy codes of the knee as well as 21060 Meniscectomy, partial or complete, temporomandibular joint (separate procedure). It is not only the knee although most definitions assume it; Meniscectmy: excision of a meniscus, usually from the knee joint.

33. a. 22510 is both unilateral and bilateral.

34. a. Fluroscopic and/or CT guidance (first paragraph under General Background)

35. d. Total disc arthroplasty: is disc replacement performed to reduce pain and disability while preserving motion. It is performed using an anterior approach.

36. c. 26508 - release of thenar muscles (e.g., thumb contracture.)

37. d. No specific code; Under code 29806 the notes state: " to report thermal capsulorhaphy, use 29999) If a surgical procedure does not match the CPT code, then DON'T code something similar or close. Code an UNLISTED procedure and then send the Operative Report with the Claim Form or it will be denied. Many unlisted codes are listed in the CPT Assistant Archives or CPT Companion booklet available from the AMA.

38. a. 2009 code.

39. b. No mention of type of lesion (Lipoma = benign) Code 23073 is correct. Don't use Quantity of 2, mailman is just extraneous information.

40. a. Description Change, 23200.

41. d. Need the correct code and MOD-RT

42. d. Note the less than 3 cm is a higher CPT Code number than the more than 3 cm. That is not typical.

43. a. In actual practice a carrier could request the -LT modifier instead of the more specific MOD-FA HCPC modifier.

44. b. Right hip, new 2010 code, subcutaneous and soft tissue.

45. b. Lots of modifiers to add to the confusion.

46. c. 28045-T2 (not T3) Should always have the fingers, toes and eyelid modifiers

47. c. No multiple quantity, Use LT MOD for left leg and new CPT code 29581.

Medical Terminology

48. d. Intra-muscular - Intra means "within" the substance of the muscle.

49. b. Kyphosis is correct. It is a forward curvature of the spine. Lordosis is convex, Scoliosis is curvature of the vertebral column, often laterally across the body.

50. c. Lordosis: Lord- "bending backward"

51. a. Skoli - a crookednes - Greek

52. b. The layers are the skin, composed of the superficial epidermis and deeper dermis, the subcutaneous tissue, the superficial fascia and then the muscle.

53. d. Arthroplasty: Either the repair of the functional power of a joint or the creation of an artificial joint.

54. b. Laminectomy: is the removal of all of the bony arch of a lamina.

55. b. Inflammation of the bone marrow and adjacent bone.

56. b. Arthrodesis is the surgical fixation or fusion of a joint. This procedure may be performed alone or in conjunction with other related procedures. When it is performed in conjunction with other procedures, it is coded in addition to the basic procedure(s) performed.

57. b. Decreased calcification of the bone

58. a. Inflammation of the bone marrow.

59. c. Excessive formation of dense, trabecular bone and calcified cartilage. Osteopetrosis is a rare congenital disorder (present at birth) in which the bones become overly dense. This results from an imbalance between the formation of bone and the breakdown of the bone.

60. d. Osteo is from the Greek "osteon", bone. A bony outgrowth or protuberance.

61. a. Grafting, reparative or plastic surgery of bones.

62. a. An asymptomatic osteosclerotic dysplasia (In English, mottled or spotted bones). Osteo is from the Greek "osteon", bone.

63. b. Atrophy of skeletal tissue.

64. b. Porous condition of the bones.

65. d. Deterioration of bone produced by ionizing radiation.

66. d. Osteorrhaphy means wiring together fragments of broken bone (suturing). Osteo is from the Greek "osteon", bone -rrhaphy to repair or reconstruct.

67. c. Abnormal hardening of bone. Osteo is from the Greek "osteon", bone. Sclerosis is hardening.

68. d. Neoplasm in bone that results in thinning and fragmentation.

69. b. Osteo-steatoma: Benign mass of the bone.

70. d. Thrombus or clotting within one or more veins of the bone.

71. d. Instrument for crushing off bits of bone.

72. a. Carpal bones, metacarpal bones and phalanges.

73. b. The largest bone of the skull, superior to the occipital bone.

74. b. There are twelve (12) ribs. I would recommend studying the vertabral column and knowing the nomenclature of the spine.

75. a. Nutrition of osseous tissue.

76. d. Laminectomy: is the removal of all of the bony arch of a lamina.

77. b. Replantation means reattaching a body part. The Replantation Codes (20802-20838) are straightforward.

78. d. Epiphyseal arrest: Also known as bone lengthening or shortening. Relating to the epiphysis, the ossification of a long bone that develops distinct from the shaft and is separated by a layer of cartilage.

79. a. An incision into the lamina.

80. d. Osteotomy: Using a saw or osteotome to cut the bone. Osteo is from the Greek "osteon", bone.

81. b. This procedure is considered neither open or closed.

82. a. Creation of a juncture between to vessels or body parts.

83. d. There are Open, Closed and Percutaneous Skeletal Fixation. These all refer to different types of fracture treatment.

84. b. The first cervical vertebra, is the Atlas. C2, the second vertebra, is the Axis.

85. d. This is a thrombus, a blood clot formed within a blood vessel and remaining attached to its place of origin, within one or more veins of the bone.

86. d. The same as reduction. It is an attempt to maneuver the bone back into proper alignment. While attaching the cast may be part of the manipulation, it is not what manipulation of a fracture means.

87. d. It can be argued that c. "Using pins, screws and an external fixation device to aid in the healing of a fracture", describes skeletal traction, it is NOT the best answer here. The question is what defines traction, which is the pulling force. Answer (C) describes skeletal traction, not the concept of traction.

88. b. A comminuted fracture is broken into several pieces.

89. d. Vertebroplasty can increase the patient's functional abilities, allow a return to the previous level of activity, and prevent further vertebral collapse. It is often used to alleviate the pain caused by a compression fracture. Typically performed on an outpatient basis, vertebroplasty is accomplished by injecting an orthopedic cement mixture through a needle into the fractured bone.

90. c. When a wound repair requires that blood vessels, tendons, or nerves be repaired, such repairs are reported using codes from the appropriate system (cardiovascular, musculoskeletal, or nervous.)

90,000 Series (medicine)

91. a. Osteopathic manipulation, acupuncture and chiropractic are all in the medicine section. But remember, just because you can coded it, does not mean you will.

92. d. General anesthesia only. Regional and local anesthesia do not apply.

93. d. 20103, ... Extremity, which would include the hand.

94. b. The fracture is reduced, or set (reduction of the fracture).

95. a. A hand was reattached through microsurgery, Replantation means "reattaching a body part". The Replantation Codes (20802-20838 are straightforward codes). Just pay attention to the body part description.

Anatomy

96. b. Chondromalacia patella is a common cause of knee cap pain or anterior knee pain. Often called Runner's Knee, this condition often affects young, otherwise healthy athletes.

97. b. Dystonia is a syndrome of sustained muscle contractions, usually producing twisting and repetitive movements or abnormal postures. With the recent mapping of genes for idiopathic torsion dystonia and identification of a gene for early onset dystonia, the description idiopathic/ primary dystonia has become outdated. It is now viewed as secondary to or symptomatic of an identified cause.

98. c. Laminotomy is an excision of a portion of a vertebral lamina in which the intervertebral foramen is enlarged by removal of a portion of the lamina. The lamina is the bone of the vertebrae.

99. d. There are thirty-three (33) vertebrae in humans, including the five

that are fused to form the sacrum (the others are separated by intervertebral discs) and the four coccygeal bones which form the tailbone. The upper three regions comprise the remaining 24, and are grouped under the names cervical (7 vertebrae), thoracic (12 vertebrae) and lumbar (5 vertebrae), according to the regions they occupy.

100. a. 27412 Autologous chondrocyte implantation, knee 27415 Osteochondral allograft, knee, open A transfusion or transplant utilizing the patient's own blood, bone marrow or tissue.

Secrets To Reducing Exam Stress

What is Stress

Stress is a normal physical response to events that make you feel threatened or upset your balance in some way, such as situations beyond your control.

The body reacts to these situations with physical, mental, and emotional responses that all merge to create what is known as stress.

When you sense danger or events beyond your control the body's defense mechanisms kick into high gear causing a built in chain reaction of events to occur. This is natural for all of us.

Remember the first time someone reprimanded you for something you had done wrong? Not necessarily a parent or relative, but someone in school or at your place of employment where you felt threatened and began feeling stressed and nervous? That was a natural reaction to a set of circumstances that caused you to feel the effects of stress.

This can be a good thing during an emergency or other event but can also be a bad thing when you are trying to concentrate or think clearly for long periods of time, such as during an exam.

What Causes Stress and Anxiety

Stress is caused by fear, plain and simple. The fear of the unknown. The fear of failing. The fear of being unprepared. The fear of loss. The fear of an uncontrollable situation.

Anything beyond our control can cause fear or a sense of danger and this causes the body to release stress hormones, thus increasing your stress and anxiety level.

There are other factors that cause stress too including family, income, job, friends, life situations and others but the main focus of this book is stress directly attributed to exam preparation and taking an exam.

Once you learn how to reduce and manage stress for an exam you can certainly expand its uses to other areas of your life as well. As a matter of fact, I highly recommend that you do. The facts are clear, the less stress you have in your life the longer you will live and the better quality of life you will have.

What Are The Side Effects Of Stress

When stress is not controlled it can cause a significant amount of problems for people taking an exam. You have likely already experienced some of the side effects of stress including:

• Memory Problems

• Lack of Concentration

• Poor Judgement

• Negative Thoughts

• Headaches

• High Blood Pressure

• Upset Stomach

Each of these side effects can affect your exam preparation efforts and performance. As a matter of fact, in some extreme cases it can cause people to "lock up" and have difficulty even taking an exam. These cases are rare but they do exist. If you suffer from this type of reaction you know all too well how difficult it is to perform under these conditions, let alone excel or perform well enough to earn a passing grade.

So how can you control or minimize the effects of stress and even make it work for you?

Learn to Relax

Setting your mind at ease and learning how to relax can reduce stress dramatically. This is much easier said than done, however, there are different techniques to help you relax and each have there own set of benefits.

There are many different ways to relax your mind and body. Some are more difficult than others. Let's begin with an easy way to reduce even the most sever cases of stress.

Slow Breathing

When you begin to feel the effects of stress your breathing accelerates and your heart rate quickens. This is caused by adrenaline being pumped into your system from the body's reaction to a circumstance or situation.

The first thing you have to do is recognize that you are experiencing stress. After you have done that, the easiest and fastest way to reduce your stress level is to slow your breathing.

If you have ever watched a sporting event you have probably seen top athletes using this method to slow their heart rate, reduce adrenaline flow, relax their muscles, and clear their minds.

This helps them think more clearly, react more rapidly, and perform at a higher level. This is exactly what you want to do.

Top athletes do this when adrenaline is not a good thing and can effect performance.

A good example of this is golf. A golfer relies heavily on muscle memory to produce accurate and consistent golf shots. When adrenaline is introduced into their system, say during the final round of a tournament, it can cause a variation in the distance they hit the ball.

This can make them inconsistent at the very time when they need to be the most consistent.

And at the same time... with the stress level now amped up it can cause a player who normally makes sound decisions to now make questionable ones. This is strikingly similar to an exam situation.

Give this method a try. Take a deep breath and exhale slowly. Repeat this several times until your muscles are totally relaxed and your heart rate slows.

Use this method before studying and prior to and during the exam itself! It will help you think more clearly and be able to recall learned information more rapidly. This technique should be the first thing you do when you start to feel anxious or stressed.

"SOMETIMES WHEN PEOPLE ARE UNDER STRESS THEY HATE TO THINK, AND IT'S THE TIME THEY MOST NEED TO THINK."

PRESIDENT BILL CLINTON

Meditation

Please don't be intimidated by the word "meditation". It is not something to fear, rather something to embrace once you know a little more about it.

Meditation can give your mind a chance to take a much needed break, to "shut down", relax and recharge.

The biggest misconception about meditation is that it is something complex. It isn't. It is simply the process of relaxing your mind and body to give it a much needed break. This is exactly what you need to relieve stress.

Time to Meditate

Meditation does not take that long to do and it can be immensely valuable for your mind, body, and spirit. Scheduling a time to meditate is the best way to make sure it happens on a regular basis.

Set aside ten minutes prior to your scheduled study time each day to meditate. This will get you into the routine of doing it. Also schedule ten to twenty minutes prior to taking an exam to meditate when possible. It will help you relax and open your mind for better memory retention during study time and better information recall during exam time.

Meditation Exercises

Follow these simple steps to enjoy a deeper sense of relaxation.

- Sit in a relaxed position.
- Close your eyes.
- Rest your hands, palms up, on your lap.
- Breathe slowly and slightly deeper than normal.

- Concentrate on your breath coming in and going out.
- Quiet your mind. If you are thinking of something try to release the thought and concentrate on breathing again.
- As you become relaxed repeat a calming word or phrase such as "I feel calm" or "I can achieve", or even "I am the best".
- After ten minutes open your eyes slowly.

This should thoroughly relax you and give you positive thoughts and energy. Now your mind is free to accept new information when studying and ready to recall learned information more rapidly and accurately when taking an exam.

Meditation is nothing more than focused relaxation for the mind and body. Look at it this way. You rest your body six to eight hours per night. Sometimes your mind is resting but not always. So your mind doesn't get as much rest as your body does, just as everything else, it needs rest to be able to perform at a high level.

This is good for daily use, but *ultra* effective prior to exam preparation and before an actual exam.

Set Up A Routine

One of the most important actions you can take to reduce stress and anxiety is set up a study routine.

By setting up a regular study routine you remove the stress of trying to find time everyday to study. Schedule the time in advance. Commit to it and stick to it.

You know what time you have to go to work everyday... right? Why not know what time you are going to study everyday? All good habits are scheduled and repeated. Study time should be no different.

Scheduling

The best time to lay out a schedule is about a month to forty five days prior to an exam when possible. All exams are different but mapping out a consistent plan is essential. This is your way to say "this is important to me".

This will give you enough time to review all the material in a timely manner without cramming it all in at the last minute. This alone will reduce your stress level significantly as well as boost your confidence.

How Often Should You Study

A good study routine should consist of regularly scheduled short periods of uninterrupted and focused study time every day. This will give you time to absorb the information when you are alert and can concentrate fully.

Your study time should not consist of hours upon hours of study time in one day and then no study time for several days. This will wear you down and reduce your ability to retain and recall information.

The last minute "all nighter" is the worst thing you can do! This time should only be for a last minute review of the most difficult material.

Plodding through hundreds of pages of information the night before an exam will only deprive you of sleep you desperately need and dilute any information you have already committed to memory.

You might occasionally "luck out" on an exam this way but keep in mind how much better you could have done had you prepared the right way.

How Long Should You Study

The ideal daily study time is an hour to two hours per day maximum! This will ultimately depend on your work, home, family, or school schedule of course but try to arrange something as close to this as possible.

If you schedule four to five hours or more in one day you are most likely defeating the purpose and wasting your time as your retention will start to decrease in hours three and beyond.

This is specially true if you have other commitments that require your time. Scheduling three or more hours of study time per day can actually add MORE stress to your life and reduce your sleeping time.

Either way this is exactly what you want to avoid at all costs! And I do mean ALL COSTS!

Scheduling time each day will keep you mentally fresh and absorbing good information PLUS it will give you the proper time for other commitments too! The outcome... reduce stressed.

Study With A Buddy

Whenever possible try to study with a buddy. Each person brings a different perspective to the learning process. This is a good way to retain new information because you are more focused on the task at hand when you are with someone else.

Plus, when you commit to study with a buddy the chances are you will actually follow through with your scheduled study time. No one likes to break a promise or commitment.

Commitment

Committing to study with a buddy is kind of like working out. It is hard to get motivated and push yourself to workout daily by yourself. That is just a fact. Only the most disciplined people can do this on their own and even some times they find it a challenge.

When you commit to meet a friend to workout it is much easier to keep your routine and commitment. Even though you may not want to workout that day, you recall the commitment you made to your friend and off you go to follow up on your commitment.

That commitment actually carries a lot of psychological weight with it. That is why people follow through with commitments made to others or in public and why it is important for you to commit to study with a buddy.

Plus the company never hurts either. Chances are you will both motivate each other to do more than you would have done alone.

The more you feel that you are not "in this alone" the more relaxed and confident you will be and the more you will get done.

Note: IMPORTANT**** *Study with a positive minded person. Don't get stuck listening to negative people and their excuses why they can't do this or that. These people are always looking to drag other people "down to their level" and are always reluctant to change to better themselves.*

If you arrange to study with a buddy and the person starts making negative comments... get out now! Don't waist your time trying to bring them up or convert them to your way of thinking.... it won't work! Stay positive and spend your time studying... not counseling. Leave that to the professionals.

Develop Your Concentration

Concentration is described as "intense mental application; complete attention".

It is your minds ability to focus on the task at hand and block out all other influences and distractions. To concentrate on one thing and one thing exclusively... the exam.

Information Retention

Your ability to concentrate is vital to your exam success. The more you concentrate on the subject materials the better you will retain and recall the information when the time comes to perform.

When you concentrate solely on the material it allows you less time to worry about other "stressors" or to give time for negative thoughts to enter in. And negative thoughts will try to work their way in. Self doubt is something that can be destructive so don't give your mind an opportunity to entertain negative thoughts.

For you to perform your best, all attention must be on the study material and the exam. This deep level of concentration will help you maximize your study time. In most cases, the better you can concentrate during your study time the less study time you will actually have to schedule. The saying "quality over quantity" applies to exam preparation too!

I mean... really, who wants to study for 5 hours at one sitting when you can study for 2 hours, with a high level of concentration and focus, and get the same results. No one. **Study Smarter, Not Longer!**

Benefits

Training your mind to concentrate on the task at hand will keep positive thoughts flowing and block out negative thoughts. Think of your mind as a bowl. You can only put so much in a bowl. So the more positive thoughts you put into the bowl the less room there is for negative ones.

Some of the benefits of increasing your level of concentration included:

• Peace of mind

• Self confidence

• Inner strength

• Ability to focus your mind

• Increased memory

• Ability to study and comprehend more quickly

• Less study time

Exercises

Here are some exercises to help you develop your concentration.

1) Select one thought and concentrate on it for ten minutes. This will be difficult at first but the more you do it the easier it will be to block out all other thoughts and concentrate on the one thought you have chosen.

2) Count the words in a paragraph. Count them again to ensure accuracy. Once you have completed this, count several paragraphs and then an entire page.

3) Take an object such as a spoon, fork, or anything out of a drawer. Try to concentrate on the object without mentally describing the object in words. Just focus on the object from all directions.

4) Draw a circle and color it in with any color. Now focus on the object and try not to think of any words, just focus on the object for several minutes.

5) Lie down and relax all your muscles. Once you are completely relaxed concentrated on your heartbeat and imagine your blood flowing throughout your body. After several minutes you should be able to feel the blood moving through your veins.

6) Watch the second hand on a clock. Focus just on the second hand and nothing else. Do this for two to three minutes and fight off the urge to let any other thoughts interfere with your concentration.

7) Close your eyes and visualize the number one. Say the number "one" in your head once you visualize it clearly. Now let it go and focus on the number two and repeat the process up to ten.

8) Take a coin out of your pocket. Relax every muscle in your body and concentrate on the coin and only the coin. View everything about it, its shape, color, material makeup nicks, words. Now close your eyes and visualize the coin in full detail. If you can not visualize the coin in full detail open your eyes and try again.

9) Sit in a chair and relax. Focus on a spot on the wall and release all other thoughts from your mind. Now while looking at the spot on the wall focus on your breathing. Breath in slowly and then exhale slowly. Do this for several minutes.

10) Read an article in the newspaper. Capture the essentials of the article. Now describe the article in as few words as possible to a friend or just aloud to yourself.

Learning to concentrate fully on the task at hand is difficult but the benefits are enormous. It is easy to let your mind wander off and loose your train of thought during an exam.

The better your concentration is during your exam preparation the better your exam scores will be. It is as simple as that.

Concentration is critical, specially towards the end of the exam when it is easy to get distracted and lose focus as you start to get tired.

This is when this training will pay off. You <u>will</u> remain focused and keep your concentration though the entire exam.

Note: IMPORTANT**** *These exercises are not for everyone, however, they are a valuable tool when learning to increase your concentration and mental focus.*

Try to do the exercises every other day. You will notice an increase in your information retention and recall. Plus this will help you study more efficiently and effectively!

Power of Positive Thinking

Positive thinking can reduce stress, improve your overall health, and make you much more interesting and fun to be around.

Although it is unclear exactly why positive thinkers experience health benefits, one of the theories is it helps them deal with stressful situations better. They are thinking of the best outcome, not the worst outcome, and this creates less stress and anxiety. This is better for the mind and the body.

I'll never forget an acquaintance of mine way back in the mid 80's who would shoot down new ideas like clay pigeons. Whenever a new idea would come up he would spend three times the intellectual effort to shoot it down than to consider if it would ever work. In his eyes "it would never work" no matter what it was.

Does that guy sound familiar to you? My guess is he probably does. You might have one or several people like this in your life right now. The best thing you can do is run... run... run.

I have nothing against shooting holes in a new idea to see if it stands the test of scrutiny, but just to dismiss a new idea because it represents change is unhealthy.

Negative people will try with all their might to bring you down. To make you surrender your positive "can do" attitude and keep them company in their pool of negativity. Don't let them!

Glass Half Full or Empty

Are you a "glass half full" or "glass half empty" type of person? Answering this question is a good way to find out if you are an optimist or a pessimist.

If you always see the good side of things (glass half full) then you are an optimist. If not, then you are a pessimist.

Optimists (or positive people) always consider the "what if it could work" side of things. They are happy and easy with a smile. They give as much positive energy as they get from others and are usually interesting and fun to be around.

An optimist is more likely to be successful too. They "will their self to victory". They tell THEMSELVES they can do something and this starts the ball of positivity and success rolling. Just as a snowball rolling down a mountain starts small, once it gains momentum there is little way to stop it.

Self Talk

Why is self talk important? Well, the mind is always thinking and creating "self-talk". Self-talk is the endless stream of thoughts that run through your head.

Self-talk is based on information, reason, logic, and prior experience. Self-talk also comes from misconceptions created because of misinformation or lack of information. This can be negative or positive, depending on your outlook.

For example, if someone asked you to jump over a hurdle and you've never jumped over a hurdle before, your mind would tell you either "you can do this" or "no way you can do this". This is commonly referred to as self-talk.

"PROGRAM THE VOICE INSIDE YOUR HEAD. IT WILL LISTEN, YOU OWN IT."

Programing your self talk will help you control the way you look at things and the attitude you have towards them. Self-talk is enormously powerful and you want to have it on your side.

A good example of the power of self-talk became apparent to me while working out several years ago and its power and control made a lasting impression on me.

In 1998 I started to lap swim at the local YMCA. I started to lap swim for several reasons. First, to lose weight that had accumulated over years of sitting behind a desk and remaining inactive. And second, to relieve some of the stress that comes with an upper level management job that I had been promoted to several years before.

The process of building up to a meaningful workout was slow at first, only a swimming a few laps per session. But over time I had built up to swimming 27 laps (which equalled 3/4 of a mile) per session.

I stayed at that level for many years, mainly because I could get my workout in over an hour long lunch break. But a funny thing happened several years ago when I finally went to work for myself. And it was all brought to light while talking to fellow lap swimmer at the local YMCA.

Through conversation she asked "how far do you swim each day". I said "3/4 of a mile". She asked, "why don't you just swim a mile"? "I don't know" I replied. "I have been doing this for years and never gave it much thought".

The next time in the pool I tried to swim a mile (36 laps) and around lap number twenty my mind began telling me I was tired and it was almost time to quit.

And sure enough, at lap twenty seven I was in no position to go any further. I was done. My mind had convinced my body that 3/4 of a mile was enough for today.

It was hard to believe that my body just started to feel exhausted around the 3/4 mile mark, knowing full well I could swim more laps. So the next day I decided to control my self-talk and tell myself "I am going to swim thirty six laps today" and "I could do anything I put my mind to". I was literally trying to trick myself into thinking I could swim a full mile.

Swimming a full mile was not a problem that day because my mind was reinforcing the belief that I could swim a mile. By controlling my self-talk and keeping the self-talk positive instead of negative I was able to control the outcome and achieve more than what my mind had previously programed me to accept as my unconscious limit.

I have also used this technique to swim two miles in one session and lose over 60 pounds. Controlling your self-talk is powerful, and it works.

Unconscious Limits

Your mind sets unconscious limits for everything that you do based on previous experience and other inputs of information such as things you read or discuss with others. Your mind processes all this information to set predetermined limits for you.

This was exceptionally powerful when world class runners were trying to break the four minute mile mark. It was generally thought that no one could ever run a mile under four minutes.

And for years no one could surpass that mark until May 6th, 1954. Sir Roger Bannister ran a mile in 3:59. Until that day no one had ever recorded running a mile under four minutes.

How strong was that unconscious limit? So strong that it only took **_46 days_** for the record to be broken. The unconscious limit had been stripped away, and in only 46 days another runner achieved what only one man had ever achieved before. The sub four minute mile.

The same applies to your exam preparation. Remove your unconscious limits and give your mind the freedom to perform the way it is capable of. Learning to channel self-talk in a positive direction can help you achieve more than you ever imagined.

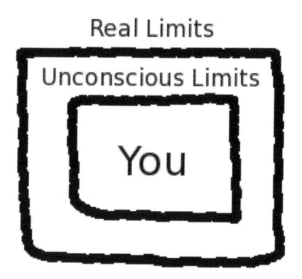

Train Your Mind

In the end, the mind will do what you <u>train</u> it to do. For example, do you ever catch yourself saying subconsciously that you *can't* do something? Of course you have. We all have. That is because we haven't trained our minds to accept the challenge of the task we want to perform.

It is our job to change the way we think. Think positive thoughts. "I CAN do this". "I am the best". "I <u>will</u> pass the exam". Train your mind to think positively and this will reduce your stress level and give you a confident feeling going into the exam.

Do not let others, or your surroundings, dictate your mental state of mind. <u>YOU</u> have the ultimate control and <u>YOU</u> control whether you think positive or negative thoughts.

This takes time and it is something that should be practiced daily. Do not think you can think positive once and everything will occur as you would like it. It just doesn't work that way. Even when you fail, resist the urge to be negative. Everything worthwhile takes some effort. But over time this will work in your favor.

You have to remember you are potentially trying to undo years of "I CAN"T" programming. Years of people telling you "YOU CAN'T" and "NO" and "IT WILL NEVER WORK".

Those are powerful messages built in to your mind. We have all heard them for many years and now is the time to turn it around.

The first "YES I CAN", and "I CAN DO WHATEVER I PUT MY MIND TO" will begin the change. It will start the little snowball rolling down the mountain... and with a little momentum comes massive change!

Self Confidence

Confidence shows in everything you do. From how you look at life to how you treat others. Confident people are people who take action. Confident people are the "doers" in the world. The people who look for ways for things to work rather than look for ways for things to fail.

Confidence is not arrogance. Confidence comes from taking decisive action and not from the outcome of that action. Confident people do not shy away from taking action because they are afraid of a failed outcome. They take action and are undaunted by the prospect of failure.

Arrogance, however, is exactly the opposite. Arrogance does not come from taking action, it comes from the result of the action. Arrogance highlights achievements and hides failures never learning anything from either.

An arrogant person is defined, in their own mind, by both their accomplishments and failures and will shy away from taking action because of the prospect of failure.

Developing Confidence

Confidence is developed through a series of "wins" or "achievements". It is developed through facing your fears and overcoming them. This gives you strength and confidence in your ability to overcome. The more you overcome, the more confident you become.

So how do you build confidence in your ability to pass an exam? Simple.... preparation! Face your fears head on and take action. Prepare every day until you know you are going to pass... there is not doubt!

Review the study material over and over again and build your level of confidence. There is no substitute for hard work and hard work builds confidence.

Have you ever seen a person walk into a room and everyone pays attention? They have a certain confidence about them that radiates form within.

They are not the wealthiest in the room. Nor the most attractive person. But this inner confidence puts them at ease when everyone else may be timid or afraid to step out of their comfort zone.

Confidence and the Exam

Your confidence will have a direct effect on your exam results. If you are confident in your ability to pass the exam it lowers your stress level and opens your mind for clearer thinking. When you project confidence your body reacts differently to circumstances. It gives you the calmness to perform at a high level.

Confidence only comes through preparation. The more you prepare, the more confident you will be in your ability to ace your exam.
This is the type of confidence you must have when you walk into the exam. An undeniable belief that you will pass the exam because of your preparation, determination, and hard work.

Nothing will stand in your way from achieving your goal!

"YOU GAIN STRENGTH, COURAGE AND CONFIDENCE BY EVERY EXPERIENCE IN WHICH YOU STOP TO LOOK FEAR IN THE FACE. YOU ARE ABLE TO SAY TO YOURSELF, 'I HAVE LIVED THROUGH THIS HORROR. I CAN TAKE THE NEXT THING THAT COMES ALONG.' YOU MUST DO THE THING YOU THINK YOU CANNOT DO."

ELEANOR ROOSEVELT

Sleep and Nutrition

The final piece of the puzzle to reducing stress is proper sleep and nutrition. Your body and mind can only function at its highest level if you give it proper rest and proper nutrition (fuel).

Your body and mind needs time to rest and good food to perform. This is easy to overlook and many times it is the first thing you sacrifice when you are preparing for an exam.

You can do everything else right to reduce stress and prepare for an exam but failing to get proper rest and nutrition could cause it all to go to waste.

Once you think about it you can see why these are essential ingredients (no pun intended) to successful exam preparation.

Sleep

Why is sleep so important? Because it is the only time your body has a chance to recharge.

A good sleep regiment should consist of at least six hours of sleep each night so your body and mind are fresh and ready to go the next morning. Anything less an you will not be fully rested and your performance will suffer because of it.

Stress can also impact sleep patterns to a point that is unhealthy. Stress related sleep disorders are fairly common and can have a major impact on your exam performance.

How many times have you tried to solve work or family related problems well into the night. Sometimes it just cannot be avoided but trying to leave work at work and going to bed with a clear mind will leave you refreshed and ready to tackle the problems of the day when the next day arrives.

To get a better nights sleep try these simple tips to reduce stress and rest up.

1) List problems bothering you with possible solutions before bed.

2) Put work into perspective. When work is over, leave it. Turn it off.

3) Designate cell free time. Even if it is only a half hour or during dinner.

4) Never check work email before bed.

5) Try to simplify one thing each day.

6) Grab a nap if you can. Sleep reduces stress hormones.

7) Laugh! Laughter reduces stress and raises <u>anti-stress</u> hormones making it easier to fall asleep.

8) Owning a pets can significantly lower your heart rate and blood pressure letting you rest longer.

9) Hug a family member. Affection reduces stress and makes it easier to sleep.

10) Take a fifteen minute walk. Exercise is the <u>BEST</u> stress reliever and you will be ready to sleep when the time comes!

These tips can make it easier to get a good nights rest and ready to go in the morning.

Nutrition

Proper nutrition to reduce stress you say? Yes, it's true! Proper nutrition plays a key role in our body's performance and ability to rest.

There is plenty of information about the ties between nutrition and sleep. One of my favorite articles is called "Sleep Deeper with Better Nutrition". It covers a mound of information about protein "super foods" and herbs that will help you get a better nights rest naturally.

Some of the "super foods" are items such as green tea, buffalo, walnuts, sardines, artichokes, kiwis, dark chocolate, cherries, and many others. These foods supply the body with super fuel and burn very efficiently so you don't feel full or tired after eating them.

I prefer making adjustments to diet over prescription drugs or other methods because it is natural and enhances the body's ability to rest.

Food or drink that contain sugar or caffeine can give you a temporary boost but the crash won't help you towards the end of the exam when you typically need it the most so try to avoid these.

What If I Fail?

The most successful people fail all the time! It is a result of taking action. There is no shame in failure, only shame in not getting back up, learning from your mistakes, and trying again.

Golf legend Jack Nicklaus used to welcome a bad golf hole or two each round because the sooner he got them out of the way the sooner he could move on and make the round a great one. He embraced temporary failure as part of being successful.

Truthfully, the more you fail the closer you are to succeeding as long as you learn from your mistakes. Few people succeed without failing many times first. It's a learning process and failure is one of the steps. You can say failure is the downpayment on success and it really is. Chances are good you will fail before you succeed but don't let it define you or hold you back. Expect it and learn from it. If you don't fail it shows you haven't taken action and just sat on the sidelines and that is the worst fate of all.

Overcome your fear of failure and success will be yours. Nothing will stand in your way. Preparation is the key. If you have prepared properly you will not fail. But if you should, embrace it, be accountable for it, and start again with more resolve than ever.

The highway is littered with people who have failed. Everyone fails. The people who win get right back on the horse and start riding again.

"I HAVE NOT FAILED. I'VE JUST FOUND 10,000 WAYS THAT WON'T WORK."

THOMAS EDISON

Getting Help

Is there a certain section of material that is just not making sense or sinking in? GET HELP! Don't wait or, worse yet, be too shy to ask for help. Search out help as fast as you can. Now is not the time to be shy or hesitate to ask for assistance.

Many teachers and instructors are more than willing to give you a helping hand. That is their profession and most of them generally love to help people. Take advantage of their help if you need it.

REMEMBER, YOU ARE NOT IN THIS ALONE!

Reaching out for help and getting it will give you a feeling of accomplishment and confidence. That confidence will be your friend and something you want to continually build upon as you ready yourself for your exam.

"ONE IMPORTANT KEY TO SUCCESS IS SELF-CONFIDENCE. AN IMPORTANT KEY TO SELF- CONFIDENCE IS PREPARATION."

ARTHUR ASHE

Common Anatomical Terminology

Anatomy terminology can seem complex and overwhelming when just starting out. Once you familiarize yourself with some of the more common terms it will make your preparation much easier. Just like anything else, it will take practice. Learn and few terms each day and before you know it you will have established a good base to work from.

Take time to familiarize yourself with these terms to make you a better medical coder.

Anatomy Terminology - Number	
Term	**Meaning**
mono-, uni-	one
bi	two
tri	three

Anatomy Terminology - Direction and Position

Term	Meaning
ab-	away from
ad-	toward
ecto-, exo-	outside
endo-	inside
epi-	upon
anterior or ventral	at or near the front surface of the body
posterior or dorsal	at or near the real surface of the body
superior	above
inferior	below
lateral	side
distal	farthest from center
proximal	nearest to center

Anatomy Terminology - Basic Terms	
Term	**Meaning**
abdominal	abdomen
buccal	cheek
cranial	skull
digital	fingers and toes
femoral	thigh
gluteal	buttocks
hallux	great toe
inguinal	groin
lumbar	lowest part of spine
mammary	breast
nasal	nose
occipital	back of head
pectoral	breastbone
thoracic	chest
umbilical	navel
ventral	belly

Anatomy Terminology - Conditions - Prefixes

Term	Meaning
ambi-	both
dys-	bad, painful, difficult
eu-	good, normal
homo-	same
iso-	equal, same
mal-	bad, poor

Anatomy Terminology - Conditions - Suffixes

Term	Meaning
-algia	pain
-emia	blood
-itis	inflammation
-lysis	destruction, breakdown
-oid	like
-opathy	disease of
-pnea	breathing

Anatomy Terminology - Surgical Procedures	
Term	**Meaning**
-centesis	puncture a cavity to remove fluid
-ectomy	surgical removal or excision
-ostomy	a new permanent opening
-otomy	cutting into, incision
-opexy	surgical fixation
-oplasty	surgical repair
-otripsy	crushing or destroying

Medical Terminology Prefix, Root, and Suffixes

Being familiar with Medical Terminology prefixes, roots and suffixes are essential for a medical coder. This illustrates how roots, prefixes, and suffixes are used to denote number or size, direction, color, anatomical locations, as well as other meanings.

Medical Terminology - Prefixes and Roots Denoting Number or Size	
Term	**Meaning**
bi-	two
dipl/o	two, double
hemi-	half
hyper-	over or more than usual
hypo-	under or less than usual
iso-	equal, same
macro-	large
megal/o-	enlargement
micro-	small
mono-	one
multi-	many
nulli-	none
poly-	many
semi-	half, partial
tri-	three
uni-	one

Medical Terminology - Roots Denoting Color	
Term	**Meaning**
chlor/o	green
cyan/o	blue
erythr/o	red
leuk/o	white
melan/o	black
xanth/o	yellow

Medical Terminology - Prefixes and Roots Denoting Relative Direction	
Term	**Meaning**
per-	through
peri-	around
post-	behind, after
poster/o	behind
pre-	before, in front of
pro-	before
retr/o	behind, in back of
sub-	under
super-	beyond
supra-	above
syn-	together
trans-	across
ventr/o	belly

Medical Terminology - Roots Denoting Anatomical Location

Term	Meaning
abdomin/o	abdomen
acr/o	extremity
aden/o	gland
angi/o	vessel
arter/i/o	artery
arthr/o	joint
blast/o	embryo
blephar/o	eyelid
bronch/i/o	bronchus
calcane/o	calaneous
cardi/o	heart
carp/o	carpal, wrist
cephal/o	head
cerebr/o	cerebrum
cheil/o	lip
chol/e	bile, gall
chondr/o	cartilage
cocc/i	coccus
col/o	colon
colp/o	vagina

Medical Terminology - Roots Denoting Anatomical Location	
Term	**Meaning**
condyl/o	condyle
core/o, cor/o	pupil
corne/o	cornea
cost/o	ribs
crani/o	cranium
cycl/o	ciliary body
cyst/o	bladder, sac
cyt/o	cell
dactyl/o	fingers or toes
dent/o	tooth
derm/o	skin
dermat/o	skin
duoden/o	duodenum
enter/o	intestine
esophag/o	esophagus
fibr/o	fiber
gangli/o	ganglion
gastr/o	stomach
gingiv/o	gums
gloss/o	tongue

Medical Terminology - Roots Denoting Anatomical Location

Term	Meaning
gynec/o	women
hem/o, hemat/o	blood
hepat/o	liver
hidr/o	sweat
humer/o	humerus
hydr/o	water
hyster/o	uterus
ile/o	ileum
irid/o, ir/o	iris
ischi/o	ischium
jejun/o	jejunum
kerat/o	cornea
lacrim/o	tear
laryng/o	larynx
lip/o	fat
lith/o	stone, calculus
lumb/o	loin, lumbar area
ment/o	chin
my/o	muscle
myel/o	spinal cord, bone marrow

Medical Terminology - Roots Denoting Anatomical Location

Term	Meaning
nas/o	nose
nephr/o	kidney
neur/o	nerve
omphal/o	umbilicus, navel
onych/o	nail
oophor/o	ovary
opthalm/o	eye
orchid/o	testicles
oste/o	bone
ot/o	ear
pancreat/o	pancreas
pely/i	pelvis
peps/o/ia	digestion
phalang/o	phalange
pharyng/o	pharynx
phas/o	speech
phleb/o	veins
pleur/o	pleura
pne/o	air, breathing
pneum/o, pneumono	lung

Medical Terminology - Roots Denoting Anatomical Location	
Term	**Meaning**
pod/o	foot
proct/o	rectum, anus
psych/o	mind
pub/o	pubis
py/o	pus
pyel/o	kidney
rect/o	rectum
ren/o	kidney
retin/o	retina
rhin/o	nose
salping/o	fallopian tube
scler/o	sclera
spermat/o	sperm
splen/o	spleen
stern/o	sternum, breastbone
stomat/o	mouth
thorac/o	thorax, chest
trache/o	trachea
traumat/o	tramua
tympan/o	eardrum

Medical Terminology - Roots Denoting Anatomical Location	
Term	**Meaning**
ur/o	urine
ureter/o	ureter
urethr/o	urethra
vas/o	vessel
viscer/o	gut, contents of the abdomen

Medical Terminology - Other Prefixes	
Term	**Meaning**
a-, an-	without
anti-	against
auto-	self
brady-	slow
con-	with
contra-	against
dis-	free of
dys-	difficult or without pain
mal-	bad, poor
neo-	new
syn-	together
tachy-	fast

Medical Terminology - Other Roots	
Term	**Meaning**
necr/o	dead
noct/i	night
par/o	bear
phag/o	eat
phil/o	attraction
plast/o	repair, formation
pyr/o	fire, fever
scler/o	tough, hard
sinistr/o	left
syphil/o	syphilis
therap/o	treatment
therm/o	heat
thromb/o	thrombosis
troph/o	development

Medical Terminology - Other Suffixes	
Term	**Meaning**
algia	pain
ar	pertaining to
centesis	puncture
clysis	irrigation
ectasia	dilatation, dilation
ectomy	excision
emes/is	vomiting
emia	blood
esthesia	feelings
genesis, gen/o	development, formation, beginning
gnosis	know
ia	noun ending
ia, ic	pertaining to
it is	inflammation
manual	hand
meter	measuring instrument
oid	resembling
ologist	one who studies
ology	study of
oma	tumor

Medical Terminology - Other Suffixes	
Term	**Meaning**
opia	vision
orrhagia	hemorrhage
orrhaphy	suture
orrhea	flow
orrhexis	rupture
osis	condition of
ostomy	new opening
otomy	incision
pedal	foot
pexy	fixing, fixation
phob/ia	fear
plasm	growth
plegia, plegic	paralysis
ptosis	drooping
scope, scopy	examining, looking at
spasm	twitching
sperm	sperm
stasis	slow, stop
tome	instrument
tripsy	crushing

Notes

Scoring Sheets
Tear out for easy use

1) A B C D
2) A B C D
3) A B C D
4) A B C D
5) A B C D
6) A B C D
7) A B C D
8) A B C D
9) A B C D
10) A B C D
11) A B C D
12) A B C D
13) A B C D
14) A B C D
15) A B C D
16) A B C D
17) A B C D
18) A B C D
19) A B C D
20) A B C D
21) A B C D
22) A B C D
23) A B C D
24) A B C D
25) A B C D
26) A B C D
27) A B C D
28) A B C D
29) A B C D

30) A B C D
31) A B C D
32) A B C D
33) A B C D
34) A B C D
35) A B C D
36) A B C D
37) A B C D
38) A B C D
39) A B C D
40) A B C D
41) A B C D
42) A B C D
43) A B C D
44) A B C D
45) A B C D
46) A B C D
47) A B C D
48) A B C D
49) A B C D
50) A B C D
51) A B C D
52) A B C D
53) A B C D
54) A B C D
55) A B C D
56) A B C D
57) A B C D
58) A B C D
59) A B C D
60) A B C D

61) A B C D
62) A B C D
63) A B C D
64) A B C D
65) A B C D
66) A B C D
67) A B C D
68) A B C D
69) A B C D
70) A B C D
71) A B C D
72) A B C D
73) A B C D
74) A B C D
75) A B C D
76) A B C D
77) A B C D
78) A B C D
79) A B C D
80) A B C D
81) A B C D
82) A B C D
83) A B C D
84) A B C D
85) A B C D
86) A B C D
87) A B C D
88) A B C D
89) A B C D
90) A B C D
91) A B C D

92)	A	B	C	D	123)	A	B	C	D
93)	A	B	C	D	124)	A	B	C	D
94)	A	B	C	D	125)	A	B	C	D
95)	A	B	C	D	126)	A	B	C	D
96)	A	B	C	D	127)	A	B	C	D
97)	A	B	C	D	128)	A	B	C	D
98)	A	B	C	D	129)	A	B	C	D
99)	A	B	C	D	130)	A	B	C	D
100)	A	B	C	D	131)	A	B	C	D
101)	A	B	C	D	132)	A	B	C	D
102)	A	B	C	D	133)	A	B	C	D
103)	A	B	C	D	134)	A	B	C	D
104)	A	B	C	D	135)	A	B	C	D
105)	A	B	C	D	136)	A	B	C	D
106)	A	B	C	D	137)	A	B	C	D
107)	A	B	C	D	138)	A	B	C	D
108)	A	B	C	D	139)	A	B	C	D
109)	A	B	C	D	140)	A	B	C	D
110)	A	B	C	D	141)	A	B	C	D
111)	A	B	C	D	142)	A	B	C	D
112)	A	B	C	D	143)	A	B	C	D
113)	A	B	C	D	144)	A	B	C	D
114)	A	B	C	D	145)	A	B	C	D
115)	A	B	C	D	146)	A	B	C	D
116)	A	B	C	D	147)	A	B	C	D
117)	A	B	C	D	148)	A	B	C	D
118)	A	B	C	D	149)	A	B	C	D
119)	A	B	C	D	150)	A	B	C	D
120)	A	B	C	D					
121)	A	B	C	D					
122)	A	B	C	D					

Scoring Sheet 2   (tear our for easy use)

1)	A	B	C	D	31)	A	B	C	D	61)	A	B	C	D
2)	A	B	C	D	32)	A	B	C	D	62)	A	B	C	D
3)	A	B	C	D	33)	A	B	C	D	63)	A	B	C	D
4)	A	B	C	D	34)	A	B	C	D	64)	A	B	C	D
5)	A	B	C	D	35)	A	B	C	D	65)	A	B	C	D
6)	A	B	C	D	36)	A	B	C	D	66)	A	B	C	D
7)	A	B	C	D	37)	A	B	C	D	67)	A	B	C	D
8)	A	B	C	D	38)	A	B	C	D	68)	A	B	C	D
9)	A	B	C	D	39)	A	B	C	D	69)	A	B	C	D
10)	A	B	C	D	40)	A	B	C	D	70)	A	B	C	D
11)	A	B	C	D	41)	A	B	C	D	71)	A	B	C	D
12)	A	B	C	D	42)	A	B	C	D	72)	A	B	C	D
13)	A	B	C	D	43)	A	B	C	D	73)	A	B	C	D
14)	A	B	C	D	44)	A	B	C	D	74)	A	B	C	D
15)	A	B	C	D	45)	A	B	C	D	75)	A	B	C	D
16)	A	B	C	D	46)	A	B	C	D	76)	A	B	C	D
17)	A	B	C	D	47)	A	B	C	D	77)	A	B	C	D
18)	A	B	C	D	48)	A	B	C	D	78)	A	B	C	D
19)	A	B	C	D	49)	A	B	C	D	79)	A	B	C	D
20)	A	B	C	D	50)	A	B	C	D	80)	A	B	C	D
21)	A	B	C	D	51)	A	B	C	D	81)	A	B	C	D
22)	A	B	C	D	52)	A	B	C	D	82)	A	B	C	D
23)	A	B	C	D	53)	A	B	C	D	83)	A	B	C	D
24)	A	B	C	D	54)	A	B	C	D	84)	A	B	C	D
25)	A	B	C	D	55)	A	B	C	D	85)	A	B	C	D
26)	A	B	C	D	56)	A	B	C	D	86)	A	B	C	D
27)	A	B	C	D	57)	A	B	C	D	87)	A	B	C	D
28)	A	B	C	D	58)	A	B	C	D	88)	A	B	C	D
29)	A	B	C	D	59)	A	B	C	D	89)	A	B	C	D
30)	A	B	C	D	60)	A	B	C	D	90)	A	B	C	D

91) A B C D	122) A B C D
92) A B C D	123) A B C D
93) A B C D	124) A B C D
94) A B C D	125) A B C D
95) A B C D	126) A B C D
96) A B C D	127) A B C D
97) A B C D	128) A B C D
98) A B C D	129) A B C D
99) A B C D	130) A B C D
100) A B C D	131) A B C D
101) A B C D	132) A B C D
102) A B C D	133) A B C D
103) A B C D	134) A B C D
104) A B C D	135) A B C D
105) A B C D	136) A B C D
106) A B C D	137) A B C D
107) A B C D	138) A B C D
108) A B C D	139) A B C D
109) A B C D	140) A B C D
110) A B C D	141) A B C D
111) A B C D	142) A B C D
112) A B C D	143) A B C D
113) A B C D	144) A B C D
114) A B C D	145) A B C D
115) A B C D	146) A B C D
116) A B C D	147) A B C D
117) A B C D	148) A B C D
118) A B C D	149) A B C D
119) A B C D	150) A B C D
120) A B C D	
121) A B C D	

Scoring Sheet 3
(tear our for easy use)

1) A B C D
2) A B C D
3) A B C D
4) A B C D
5) A B C D
6) A B C D
7) A B C D
8) A B C D
9) A B C D
10) A B C D
11) A B C D
12) A B C D
13) A B C D
14) A B C D
15) A B C D
16) A B C D
17) A B C D
18) A B C D
19) A B C D
20) A B C D
21) A B C D
22) A B C D
23) A B C D
24) A B C D
25) A B C D
26) A B C D
27) A B C D
28) A B C D

29) A B C D
30) A B C D
31) A B C D
32) A B C D
33) A B C D
34) A B C D
35) A B C D
36) A B C D
37) A B C D
38) A B C D
39) A B C D
40) A B C D
41) A B C D
42) A B C D
43) A B C D
44) A B C D
45) A B C D
46) A B C D
47) A B C D
48) A B C D
49) A B C D
50) A B C D
51) A B C D
52) A B C D
53) A B C D
54) A B C D
55) A B C D
56) A B C D
57) A B C D
58) A B C D
59) A B C D

60) A B C D
61) A B C D
62) A B C D
63) A B C D
64) A B C D
65) A B C D
66) A B C D
67) A B C D
68) A B C D
69) A B C D
70) A B C D
71) A B C D
72) A B C D
73) A B C D
74) A B C D
75) A B C D
76) A B C D
77) A B C D
78) A B C D
79) A B C D
80) A B C D
81) A B C D
82) A B C D
83) A B C D
84) A B C D
85) A B C D
86) A B C D
87) A B C D
88) A B C D
89) A B C D
90) A B C D

91)	A	B	C	D		122)	A	B	C	D
92)	A	B	C	D		123)	A	B	C	D
93)	A	B	C	D		124)	A	B	C	D
94)	A	B	C	D		125)	A	B	C	D
95)	A	B	C	D		126)	A	B	C	D
96)	A	B	C	D		127)	A	B	C	D
97)	A	B	C	D		128)	A	B	C	D
98)	A	B	C	D		129)	A	B	C	D
99)	A	B	C	D		130)	A	B	C	D
100)	A	B	C	D		131)	A	B	C	D
101)	A	B	C	D		132)	A	B	C	D
102)	A	B	C	D		133)	A	B	C	D
103)	A	B	C	D		134)	A	B	C	D
104)	A	B	C	D		135)	A	B	C	D
105)	A	B	C	D		136)	A	B	C	D
106)	A	B	C	D		137)	A	B	C	D
107)	A	B	C	D		138)	A	B	C	D
108)	A	B	C	D		139)	A	B	C	D
109)	A	B	C	D		140)	A	B	C	D
110)	A	B	C	D		141)	A	B	C	D
111)	A	B	C	D		142)	A	B	C	D
112)	A	B	C	D		143)	A	B	C	D
113)	A	B	C	D		144)	A	B	C	D
114)	A	B	C	D		145)	A	B	C	D
115)	A	B	C	D		146)	A	B	C	D
116)	A	B	C	D		147)	A	B	C	D
117)	A	B	C	D		148)	A	B	C	D
118)	A	B	C	D		149)	A	B	C	D
119)	A	B	C	D		150)	A	B	C	D
120)	A	B	C	D						
121)	A	B	C	D						

Scoring Sheet 4
(tear our for easy use)

1) A B C D
2) A B C D
3) A B C D
4) A B C D
5) A B C D
6) A B C D
7) A B C D
8) A B C D
9) A B C D
10) A B C D
11) A B C D
12) A B C D
13) A B C D
14) A B C D
15) A B C D
16) A B C D
17) A B C D
18) A B C D
19) A B C D
20) A B C D
21) A B C D
22) A B C D
23) A B C D
24) A B C D
25) A B C D
26) A B C D
27) A B C D
28) A B C D

29) A B C D
30) A B C D
31) A B C D
32) A B C D
33) A B C D
34) A B C D
35) A B C D
36) A B C D
37) A B C D
38) A B C D
39) A B C D
40) A B C D
41) A B C D
42) A B C D
43) A B C D
44) A B C D
45) A B C D
46) A B C D
47) A B C D
48) A B C D
49) A B C D
50) A B C D
51) A B C D
52) A B C D
53) A B C D
54) A B C D
55) A B C D
56) A B C D
57) A B C D
58) A B C D
59) A B C D

60) A B C D
61) A B C D
62) A B C D
63) A B C D
64) A B C D
65) A B C D
66) A B C D
67) A B C D
68) A B C D
69) A B C D
70) A B C D
71) A B C D
72) A B C D
73) A B C D
74) A B C D
75) A B C D
76) A B C D
77) A B C D
78) A B C D
79) A B C D
80) A B C D
81) A B C D
82) A B C D
83) A B C D
84) A B C D
85) A B C D
86) A B C D
87) A B C D
88) A B C D
89) A B C D
90) A B C D

91)	A	B	C	D
92)	A	B	C	D
93)	A	B	C	D
94)	A	B	C	D
95)	A	B	C	D
96)	A	B	C	D
97)	A	B	C	D
98)	A	B	C	D
99)	A	B	C	D
100)	A	B	C	D
101)	A	B	C	D
102)	A	B	C	D
103)	A	B	C	D
104)	A	B	C	D
105)	A	B	C	D
106)	A	B	C	D
107)	A	B	C	D
108)	A	B	C	D
109)	A	B	C	D
110)	A	B	C	D
111)	A	B	C	D
112)	A	B	C	D
113)	A	B	C	D
114)	A	B	C	D
115)	A	B	C	D
116)	A	B	C	D
117)	A	B	C	D
118)	A	B	C	D
119)	A	B	C	D
120)	A	B	C	D
121)	A	B	C	D

122)	A	B	C	D
123)	A	B	C	D
124)	A	B	C	D
125)	A	B	C	D
126)	A	B	C	D
127)	A	B	C	D
128)	A	B	C	D
129)	A	B	C	D
130)	A	B	C	D
131)	A	B	C	D
132)	A	B	C	D
133)	A	B	C	D
134)	A	B	C	D
135)	A	B	C	D
136)	A	B	C	D
137)	A	B	C	D
138)	A	B	C	D
139)	A	B	C	D
140)	A	B	C	D
141)	A	B	C	D
142)	A	B	C	D
143)	A	B	C	D
144)	A	B	C	D
145)	A	B	C	D
146)	A	B	C	D
147)	A	B	C	D
148)	A	B	C	D
149)	A	B	C	D
150)	A	B	C	D

Scoring Sheet 5
(tear our for easy use)

1)	A	B	C	D	29)	A	B	C	D	60)	A	B	C	D
2)	A	B	C	D	30)	A	B	C	D	61)	A	B	C	D
3)	A	B	C	D	31)	A	B	C	D	62)	A	B	C	D
4)	A	B	C	D	32)	A	B	C	D	63)	A	B	C	D
5)	A	B	C	D	33)	A	B	C	D	64)	A	B	C	D
6)	A	B	C	D	34)	A	B	C	D	65)	A	B	C	D
7)	A	B	C	D	35)	A	B	C	D	66)	A	B	C	D
8)	A	B	C	D	36)	A	B	C	D	67)	A	B	C	D
9)	A	B	C	D	37)	A	B	C	D	68)	A	B	C	D
10)	A	B	C	D	38)	A	B	C	D	69)	A	B	C	D
11)	A	B	C	D	39)	A	B	C	D	70)	A	B	C	D
12)	A	B	C	D	40)	A	B	C	D	71)	A	B	C	D
13)	A	B	C	D	41)	A	B	C	D	72)	A	B	C	D
14)	A	B	C	D	42)	A	B	C	D	73)	A	B	C	D
15)	A	B	C	D	43)	A	B	C	D	74)	A	B	C	D
16)	A	B	C	D	44)	A	B	C	D	75)	A	B	C	D
17)	A	B	C	D	45)	A	B	C	D	76)	A	B	C	D
18)	A	B	C	D	46)	A	B	C	D	77)	A	B	C	D
19)	A	B	C	D	47)	A	B	C	D	78)	A	B	C	D
20)	A	B	C	D	48)	A	B	C	D	79)	A	B	C	D
21)	A	B	C	D	49)	A	B	C	D	80)	A	B	C	D
22)	A	B	C	D	50)	A	B	C	D	81)	A	B	C	D
23)	A	B	C	D	51)	A	B	C	D	82)	A	B	C	D
24)	A	B	C	D	52)	A	B	C	D	83)	A	B	C	D
25)	A	B	C	D	53)	A	B	C	D	84)	A	B	C	D
26)	A	B	C	D	54)	A	B	C	D	85)	A	B	C	D
27)	A	B	C	D	55)	A	B	C	D	86)	A	B	C	D
28)	A	B	C	D	56)	A	B	C	D	87)	A	B	C	D
					57)	A	B	C	D	88)	A	B	C	D
					58)	A	B	C	D	89)	A	B	C	D
					59)	A	B	C	D	90)	A	B	C	D

91)	A	B	C	D	122)	A	B	C	D
92)	A	B	C	D	123)	A	B	C	D
93)	A	B	C	D	124)	A	B	C	D
94)	A	B	C	D	125)	A	B	C	D
95)	A	B	C	D	126)	A	B	C	D
96)	A	B	C	D	127)	A	B	C	D
97)	A	B	C	D	128)	A	B	C	D
98)	A	B	C	D	129)	A	B	C	D
99)	A	B	C	D	130)	A	B	C	D
100)	A	B	C	D	131)	A	B	C	D
101)	A	B	C	D	132)	A	B	C	D
102)	A	B	C	D	133)	A	B	C	D
103)	A	B	C	D	134)	A	B	C	D
104)	A	B	C	D	135)	A	B	C	D
105)	A	B	C	D	136)	A	B	C	D
106)	A	B	C	D	137)	A	B	C	D
107)	A	B	C	D	138)	A	B	C	D
108)	A	B	C	D	139)	A	B	C	D
109)	A	B	C	D	140)	A	B	C	D
110)	A	B	C	D	141)	A	B	C	D
111)	A	B	C	D	142)	A	B	C	D
112)	A	B	C	D	143)	A	B	C	D
113)	A	B	C	D	144)	A	B	C	D
114)	A	B	C	D	145)	A	B	C	D
115)	A	B	C	D	146)	A	B	C	D
116)	A	B	C	D	147)	A	B	C	D
117)	A	B	C	D	148)	A	B	C	D
118)	A	B	C	D	149)	A	B	C	D
119)	A	B	C	D	150)	A	B	C	D
120)	A	B	C	D					
121)	A	B	C	D					

Scoring Sheet 6
(tear our for easy use)

1) A B C D
2) A B C D
3) A B C D
4) A B C D
5) A B C D
6) A B C D
7) A B C D
8) A B C D
9) A B C D
10) A B C D
11) A B C D
12) A B C D
13) A B C D
14) A B C D
15) A B C D
16) A B C D
17) A B C D
18) A B C D
19) A B C D
20) A B C D
21) A B C D
22) A B C D
23) A B C D
24) A B C D
25) A B C D
26) A B C D
27) A B C D
28) A B C D

29) A B C D
30) A B C D
31) A B C D
32) A B C D
33) A B C D
34) A B C D
35) A B C D
36) A B C D
37) A B C D
38) A B C D
39) A B C D
40) A B C D
41) A B C D
42) A B C D
43) A B C D
44) A B C D
45) A B C D
46) A B C D
47) A B C D
48) A B C D
49) A B C D
50) A B C D
51) A B C D
52) A B C D
53) A B C D
54) A B C D
55) A B C D
56) A B C D
57) A B C D
58) A B C D
59) A B C D

60) A B C D
61) A B C D
62) A B C D
63) A B C D
64) A B C D
65) A B C D
66) A B C D
67) A B C D
68) A B C D
69) A B C D
70) A B C D
71) A B C D
72) A B C D
73) A B C D
74) A B C D
75) A B C D
76) A B C D
77) A B C D
78) A B C D
79) A B C D
80) A B C D
81) A B C D
82) A B C D
83) A B C D
84) A B C D
85) A B C D
86) A B C D
87) A B C D
88) A B C D
89) A B C D
90) A B C D

91)	A	B	C	D	122)	A	B	C	D
92)	A	B	C	D	123)	A	B	C	D
93)	A	B	C	D	124)	A	B	C	D
94)	A	B	C	D	125)	A	B	C	D
95)	A	B	C	D	126)	A	B	C	D
96)	A	B	C	D	127)	A	B	C	D
97)	A	B	C	D	128)	A	B	C	D
98)	A	B	C	D	129)	A	B	C	D
99)	A	B	C	D	130)	A	B	C	D
100)	A	B	C	D	131)	A	B	C	D
101)	A	B	C	D	132)	A	B	C	D
102)	A	B	C	D	133)	A	B	C	D
103)	A	B	C	D	134)	A	B	C	D
104)	A	B	C	D	135)	A	B	C	D
105)	A	B	C	D	136)	A	B	C	D
106)	A	B	C	D	137)	A	B	C	D
107)	A	B	C	D	138)	A	B	C	D
108)	A	B	C	D	139)	A	B	C	D
109)	A	B	C	D	140)	A	B	C	D
110)	A	B	C	D	141)	A	B	C	D
111)	A	B	C	D	142)	A	B	C	D
112)	A	B	C	D	143)	A	B	C	D
113)	A	B	C	D	144)	A	B	C	D
114)	A	B	C	D	145)	A	B	C	D
115)	A	B	C	D	146)	A	B	C	D
116)	A	B	C	D	147)	A	B	C	D
117)	A	B	C	D	148)	A	B	C	D
118)	A	B	C	D	149)	A	B	C	D
119)	A	B	C	D	150)	A	B	C	D
120)	A	B	C	D					
121)	A	B	C	D					

Scoring Sheet 7
(tear our for easy use)

1) A   B   C   D
2) A   B   C   D
3) A   B   C   D
4) A   B   C   D
5) A   B   C   D
6) A   B   C   D
7) A   B   C   D
8) A   B   C   D
9) A   B   C   D
10) A   B   C   D
11) A   B   C   D
12) A   B   C   D
13) A   B   C   D
14) A   B   C   D
15) A   B   C   D
16) A   B   C   D
17) A   B   C   D
18) A   B   C   D
19) A   B   C   D
20) A   B   C   D
21) A   B   C   D
22) A   B   C   D
23) A   B   C   D
24) A   B   C   D
25) A   B   C   D
26) A   B   C   D
27) A   B   C   D
28) A   B   C   D

29) A   B   C   D
30) A   B   C   D
31) A   B   C   D
32) A   B   C   D
33) A   B   C   D
34) A   B   C   D
35) A   B   C   D
36) A   B   C   D
37) A   B   C   D
38) A   B   C   D
39) A   B   C   D
40) A   B   C   D
41) A   B   C   D
42) A   B   C   D
43) A   B   C   D
44) A   B   C   D
45) A   B   C   D
46) A   B   C   D
47) A   B   C   D
48) A   B   C   D
49) A   B   C   D
50) A   B   C   D
51) A   B   C   D
52) A   B   C   D
53) A   B   C   D
54) A   B   C   D
55) A   B   C   D
56) A   B   C   D
57) A   B   C   D
58) A   B   C   D
59) A   B   C   D

60) A   B   C   D
61) A   B   C   D
62) A   B   C   D
63) A   B   C   D
64) A   B   C   D
65) A   B   C   D
66) A   B   C   D
67) A   B   C   D
68) A   B   C   D
69) A   B   C   D
70) A   B   C   D
71) A   B   C   D
72) A   B   C   D
73) A   B   C   D
74) A   B   C   D
75) A   B   C   D
76) A   B   C   D
77) A   B   C   D
78) A   B   C   D
79) A   B   C   D
80) A   B   C   D
81) A   B   C   D
82) A   B   C   D
83) A   B   C   D
84) A   B   C   D
85) A   B   C   D
86) A   B   C   D
87) A   B   C   D
88) A   B   C   D
89) A   B   C   D
90) A   B   C   D

91)	A	B	C	D	122)	A	B	C	D
92)	A	B	C	D	123)	A	B	C	D
93)	A	B	C	D	124)	A	B	C	D
94)	A	B	C	D	125)	A	B	C	D
95)	A	B	C	D	126)	A	B	C	D
96)	A	B	C	D	127)	A	B	C	D
97)	A	B	C	D	128)	A	B	C	D
98)	A	B	C	D	129)	A	B	C	D
99)	A	B	C	D	130)	A	B	C	D
100)	A	B	C	D	131)	A	B	C	D
101)	A	B	C	D	132)	A	B	C	D
102)	A	B	C	D	133)	A	B	C	D
103)	A	B	C	D	134)	A	B	C	D
104)	A	B	C	D	135)	A	B	C	D
105)	A	B	C	D	136)	A	B	C	D
106)	A	B	C	D	137)	A	B	C	D
107)	A	B	C	D	138)	A	B	C	D
108)	A	B	C	D	139)	A	B	C	D
109)	A	B	C	D	140)	A	B	C	D
110)	A	B	C	D	141)	A	B	C	D
111)	A	B	C	D	142)	A	B	C	D
112)	A	B	C	D	143)	A	B	C	D
113)	A	B	C	D	144)	A	B	C	D
114)	A	B	C	D	145)	A	B	C	D
115)	A	B	C	D	146)	A	B	C	D
116)	A	B	C	D	147)	A	B	C	D
117)	A	B	C	D	148)	A	B	C	D
118)	A	B	C	D	149)	A	B	C	D
119)	A	B	C	D	150)	A	B	C	D
120)	A	B	C	D					
121)	A	B	C	D					

Scoring Sheet 8
(tear our for easy use)

1)	A	B	C	D	29)	A	B	C	D	60)	A	B	C	D
2)	A	B	C	D	30)	A	B	C	D	61)	A	B	C	D
3)	A	B	C	D	31)	A	B	C	D	62)	A	B	C	D
4)	A	B	C	D	32)	A	B	C	D	63)	A	B	C	D
5)	A	B	C	D	33)	A	B	C	D	64)	A	B	C	D
6)	A	B	C	D	34)	A	B	C	D	65)	A	B	C	D
7)	A	B	C	D	35)	A	B	C	D	66)	A	B	C	D
8)	A	B	C	D	36)	A	B	C	D	67)	A	B	C	D
9)	A	B	C	D	37)	A	B	C	D	68)	A	B	C	D
10)	A	B	C	D	38)	A	B	C	D	69)	A	B	C	D
11)	A	B	C	D	39)	A	B	C	D	70)	A	B	C	D
12)	A	B	C	D	40)	A	B	C	D	71)	A	B	C	D
13)	A	B	C	D	41)	A	B	C	D	72)	A	B	C	D
14)	A	B	C	D	42)	A	B	C	D	73)	A	B	C	D
15)	A	B	C	D	43)	A	B	C	D	74)	A	B	C	D
16)	A	B	C	D	44)	A	B	C	D	75)	A	B	C	D
17)	A	B	C	D	45)	A	B	C	D	76)	A	B	C	D
18)	A	B	C	D	46)	A	B	C	D	77)	A	B	C	D
19)	A	B	C	D	47)	A	B	C	D	78)	A	B	C	D
20)	A	B	C	D	48)	A	B	C	D	79)	A	B	C	D
21)	A	B	C	D	49)	A	B	C	D	80)	A	B	C	D
22)	A	B	C	D	50)	A	B	C	D	81)	A	B	C	D
23)	A	B	C	D	51)	A	B	C	D	82)	A	B	C	D
24)	A	B	C	D	52)	A	B	C	D	83)	A	B	C	D
25)	A	B	C	D	53)	A	B	C	D	84)	A	B	C	D
26)	A	B	C	D	54)	A	B	C	D	85)	A	B	C	D
27)	A	B	C	D	55)	A	B	C	D	86)	A	B	C	D
28)	A	B	C	D	56)	A	B	C	D	87)	A	B	C	D
					57)	A	B	C	D	88)	A	B	C	D
					58)	A	B	C	D	89)	A	B	C	D
					59)	A	B	C	D	90)	A	B	C	D

91)	A	B	C	D	122)	A	B	C	D
92)	A	B	C	D	123)	A	B	C	D
93)	A	B	C	D	124)	A	B	C	D
94)	A	B	C	D	125)	A	B	C	D
95)	A	B	C	D	126)	A	B	C	D
96)	A	B	C	D	127)	A	B	C	D
97)	A	B	C	D	128)	A	B	C	D
98)	A	B	C	D	129)	A	B	C	D
99)	A	B	C	D	130)	A	B	C	D
100)	A	B	C	D	131)	A	B	C	D
101)	A	B	C	D	132)	A	B	C	D
102)	A	B	C	D	133)	A	B	C	D
103)	A	B	C	D	134)	A	B	C	D
104)	A	B	C	D	135)	A	B	C	D
105)	A	B	C	D	136)	A	B	C	D
106)	A	B	C	D	137)	A	B	C	D
107)	A	B	C	D	138)	A	B	C	D
108)	A	B	C	D	139)	A	B	C	D
109)	A	B	C	D	140)	A	B	C	D
110)	A	B	C	D	141)	A	B	C	D
111)	A	B	C	D	142)	A	B	C	D
112)	A	B	C	D	143)	A	B	C	D
113)	A	B	C	D	144)	A	B	C	D
114)	A	B	C	D	145)	A	B	C	D
115)	A	B	C	D	146)	A	B	C	D
116)	A	B	C	D	147)	A	B	C	D
117)	A	B	C	D	148)	A	B	C	D
118)	A	B	C	D	149)	A	B	C	D
119)	A	B	C	D	150)	A	B	C	D
120)	A	B	C	D					
121)	A	B	C	D					

Scoring Sheet 9
(tear our for easy use)

1) A B C D
2) A B C D
3) A B C D
4) A B C D
5) A B C D
6) A B C D
7) A B C D
8) A B C D
9) A B C D
10) A B C D
11) A B C D
12) A B C D
13) A B C D
14) A B C D
15) A B C D
16) A B C D
17) A B C D
18) A B C D
19) A B C D
20) A B C D
21) A B C D
22) A B C D
23) A B C D
24) A B C D
25) A B C D
26) A B C D
27) A B C D
28) A B C D

29) A B C D
30) A B C D
31) A B C D
32) A B C D
33) A B C D
34) A B C D
35) A B C D
36) A B C D
37) A B C D
38) A B C D
39) A B C D
40) A B C D
41) A B C D
42) A B C D
43) A B C D
44) A B C D
45) A B C D
46) A B C D
47) A B C D
48) A B C D
49) A B C D
50) A B C D
51) A B C D
52) A B C D
53) A B C D
54) A B C D
55) A B C D
56) A B C D
57) A B C D
58) A B C D
59) A B C D

60) A B C D
61) A B C D
62) A B C D
63) A B C D
64) A B C D
65) A B C D
66) A B C D
67) A B C D
68) A B C D
69) A B C D
70) A B C D
71) A B C D
72) A B C D
73) A B C D
74) A B C D
75) A B C D
76) A B C D
77) A B C D
78) A B C D
79) A B C D
80) A B C D
81) A B C D
82) A B C D
83) A B C D
84) A B C D
85) A B C D
86) A B C D
87) A B C D
88) A B C D
89) A B C D
90) A B C D

91)	A	B	C	D	122)	A	B	C	D
92)	A	B	C	D	123)	A	B	C	D
93)	A	B	C	D	124)	A	B	C	D
94)	A	B	C	D	125)	A	B	C	D
95)	A	B	C	D	126)	A	B	C	D
96)	A	B	C	D	127)	A	B	C	D
97)	A	B	C	D	128)	A	B	C	D
98)	A	B	C	D	129)	A	B	C	D
99)	A	B	C	D	130)	A	B	C	D
100)	A	B	C	D	131)	A	B	C	D
101)	A	B	C	D	132)	A	B	C	D
102)	A	B	C	D	133)	A	B	C	D
103)	A	B	C	D	134)	A	B	C	D
104)	A	B	C	D	135)	A	B	C	D
105)	A	B	C	D	136)	A	B	C	D
106)	A	B	C	D	137)	A	B	C	D
107)	A	B	C	D	138)	A	B	C	D
108)	A	B	C	D	139)	A	B	C	D
109)	A	B	C	D	140)	A	B	C	D
110)	A	B	C	D	141)	A	B	C	D
111)	A	B	C	D	142)	A	B	C	D
112)	A	B	C	D	143)	A	B	C	D
113)	A	B	C	D	144)	A	B	C	D
114)	A	B	C	D	145)	A	B	C	D
115)	A	B	C	D	146)	A	B	C	D
116)	A	B	C	D	147)	A	B	C	D
117)	A	B	C	D	148)	A	B	C	D
118)	A	B	C	D	149)	A	B	C	D
119)	A	B	C	D	150)	A	B	C	D
120)	A	B	C	D					
121)	A	B	C	D					

Scoring Sheet 10
(tear our for easy use)

1)	A	B	C	D
2)	A	B	C	D
3)	A	B	C	D
4)	A	B	C	D
5)	A	B	C	D
6)	A	B	C	D
7)	A	B	C	D
8)	A	B	C	D
9)	A	B	C	D
10)	A	B	C	D
11)	A	B	C	D
12)	A	B	C	D
13)	A	B	C	D
14)	A	B	C	D
15)	A	B	C	D
16)	A	B	C	D
17)	A	B	C	D
18)	A	B	C	D
19)	A	B	C	D
20)	A	B	C	D
21)	A	B	C	D
22)	A	B	C	D
23)	A	B	C	D
24)	A	B	C	D
25)	A	B	C	D
26)	A	B	C	D
27)	A	B	C	D
28)	A	B	C	D
29)	A	B	C	D
30)	A	B	C	D
31)	A	B	C	D
32)	A	B	C	D
33)	A	B	C	D
34)	A	B	C	D
35)	A	B	C	D
36)	A	B	C	D
37)	A	B	C	D
38)	A	B	C	D
39)	A	B	C	D
40)	A	B	C	D
41)	A	B	C	D
42)	A	B	C	D
43)	A	B	C	D
44)	A	B	C	D
45)	A	B	C	D
46)	A	B	C	D
47)	A	B	C	D
48)	A	B	C	D
49)	A	B	C	D
50)	A	B	C	D
51)	A	B	C	D
52)	A	B	C	D
53)	A	B	C	D
54)	A	B	C	D
55)	A	B	C	D
56)	A	B	C	D
57)	A	B	C	D
58)	A	B	C	D
59)	A	B	C	D
60)	A	B	C	D
61)	A	B	C	D
62)	A	B	C	D
63)	A	B	C	D
64)	A	B	C	D
65)	A	B	C	D
66)	A	B	C	D
67)	A	B	C	D
68)	A	B	C	D
69)	A	B	C	D
70)	A	B	C	D
71)	A	B	C	D
72)	A	B	C	D
73)	A	B	C	D
74)	A	B	C	D
75)	A	B	C	D
76)	A	B	C	D
77)	A	B	C	D
78)	A	B	C	D
79)	A	B	C	D
80)	A	B	C	D
81)	A	B	C	D
82)	A	B	C	D
83)	A	B	C	D
84)	A	B	C	D
85)	A	B	C	D
86)	A	B	C	D
87)	A	B	C	D
88)	A	B	C	D
89)	A	B	C	D
90)	A	B	C	D

91)	A	B	C	D	122)	A	B	C	D
92)	A	B	C	D	123)	A	B	C	D
93)	A	B	C	D	124)	A	B	C	D
94)	A	B	C	D	125)	A	B	C	D
95)	A	B	C	D	126)	A	B	C	D
96)	A	B	C	D	127)	A	B	C	D
97)	A	B	C	D	128)	A	B	C	D
98)	A	B	C	D	129)	A	B	C	D
99)	A	B	C	D	130)	A	B	C	D
100)	A	B	C	D	131)	A	B	C	D
101)	A	B	C	D	132)	A	B	C	D
102)	A	B	C	D	133)	A	B	C	D
103)	A	B	C	D	134)	A	B	C	D
104)	A	B	C	D	135)	A	B	C	D
105)	A	B	C	D	136)	A	B	C	D
106)	A	B	C	D	137)	A	B	C	D
107)	A	B	C	D	138)	A	B	C	D
108)	A	B	C	D	139)	A	B	C	D
109)	A	B	C	D	140)	A	B	C	D
110)	A	B	C	D	141)	A	B	C	D
111)	A	B	C	D	142)	A	B	C	D
112)	A	B	C	D	143)	A	B	C	D
113)	A	B	C	D	144)	A	B	C	D
114)	A	B	C	D	145)	A	B	C	D
115)	A	B	C	D	146)	A	B	C	D
116)	A	B	C	D	147)	A	B	C	D
117)	A	B	C	D	148)	A	B	C	D
118)	A	B	C	D	149)	A	B	C	D
119)	A	B	C	D	150)	A	B	C	D
120)	A	B	C	D					
121)	A	B	C	D					

Scoring Sheet 11
(tear our for easy use)

1)	A	B	C	D	29)	A	B	C	D	60)	A	B	C	D
2)	A	B	C	D	30)	A	B	C	D	61)	A	B	C	D
3)	A	B	C	D	31)	A	B	C	D	62)	A	B	C	D
4)	A	B	C	D	32)	A	B	C	D	63)	A	B	C	D
5)	A	B	C	D	33)	A	B	C	D	64)	A	B	C	D
6)	A	B	C	D	34)	A	B	C	D	65)	A	B	C	D
7)	A	B	C	D	35)	A	B	C	D	66)	A	B	C	D
8)	A	B	C	D	36)	A	B	C	D	67)	A	B	C	D
9)	A	B	C	D	37)	A	B	C	D	68)	A	B	C	D
10)	A	B	C	D	38)	A	B	C	D	69)	A	B	C	D
11)	A	B	C	D	39)	A	B	C	D	70)	A	B	C	D
12)	A	B	C	D	40)	A	B	C	D	71)	A	B	C	D
13)	A	B	C	D	41)	A	B	C	D	72)	A	B	C	D
14)	A	B	C	D	42)	A	B	C	D	73)	A	B	C	D
15)	A	B	C	D	43)	A	B	C	D	74)	A	B	C	D
16)	A	B	C	D	44)	A	B	C	D	75)	A	B	C	D
17)	A	B	C	D	45)	A	B	C	D	76)	A	B	C	D
18)	A	B	C	D	46)	A	B	C	D	77)	A	B	C	D
19)	A	B	C	D	47)	A	B	C	D	78)	A	B	C	D
20)	A	B	C	D	48)	A	B	C	D	79)	A	B	C	D
21)	A	B	C	D	49)	A	B	C	D	80)	A	B	C	D
22)	A	B	C	D	50)	A	B	C	D	81)	A	B	C	D
23)	A	B	C	D	51)	A	B	C	D	82)	A	B	C	D
24)	A	B	C	D	52)	A	B	C	D	83)	A	B	C	D
25)	A	B	C	D	53)	A	B	C	D	84)	A	B	C	D
26)	A	B	C	D	54)	A	B	C	D	85)	A	B	C	D
27)	A	B	C	D	55)	A	B	C	D	86)	A	B	C	D
28)	A	B	C	D	56)	A	B	C	D	87)	A	B	C	D
					57)	A	B	C	D	88)	A	B	C	D
					58)	A	B	C	D	89)	A	B	C	D
					59)	A	B	C	D	90)	A	B	C	D

91)	A	B	C	D	122)	A	B	C	D
92)	A	B	C	D	123)	A	B	C	D
93)	A	B	C	D	124)	A	B	C	D
94)	A	B	C	D	125)	A	B	C	D
95)	A	B	C	D	126)	A	B	C	D
96)	A	B	C	D	127)	A	B	C	D
97)	A	B	C	D	128)	A	B	C	D
98)	A	B	C	D	129)	A	B	C	D
99)	A	B	C	D	130)	A	B	C	D
100)	A	B	C	D	131)	A	B	C	D
101)	A	B	C	D	132)	A	B	C	D
102)	A	B	C	D	133)	A	B	C	D
103)	A	B	C	D	134)	A	B	C	D
104)	A	B	C	D	135)	A	B	C	D
105)	A	B	C	D	136)	A	B	C	D
106)	A	B	C	D	137)	A	B	C	D
107)	A	B	C	D	138)	A	B	C	D
108)	A	B	C	D	139)	A	B	C	D
109)	A	B	C	D	140)	A	B	C	D
110)	A	B	C	D	141)	A	B	C	D
111)	A	B	C	D	142)	A	B	C	D
112)	A	B	C	D	143)	A	B	C	D
113)	A	B	C	D	144)	A	B	C	D
114)	A	B	C	D	145)	A	B	C	D
115)	A	B	C	D	146)	A	B	C	D
116)	A	B	C	D	147)	A	B	C	D
117)	A	B	C	D	148)	A	B	C	D
118)	A	B	C	D	149)	A	B	C	D
119)	A	B	C	D	150)	A	B	C	D
120)	A	B	C	D					
121)	A	B	C	D					

Scoring Sheet 12
(tear our for easy use)

1)	A	B	C	D	29)	A	B	C	D	60)	A	B	C	D
2)	A	B	C	D	30)	A	B	C	D	61)	A	B	C	D
3)	A	B	C	D	31)	A	B	C	D	62)	A	B	C	D
4)	A	B	C	D	32)	A	B	C	D	63)	A	B	C	D
5)	A	B	C	D	33)	A	B	C	D	64)	A	B	C	D
6)	A	B	C	D	34)	A	B	C	D	65)	A	B	C	D
7)	A	B	C	D	35)	A	B	C	D	66)	A	B	C	D
8)	A	B	C	D	36)	A	B	C	D	67)	A	B	C	D
9)	A	B	C	D	37)	A	B	C	D	68)	A	B	C	D
10)	A	B	C	D	38)	A	B	C	D	69)	A	B	C	D
11)	A	B	C	D	39)	A	B	C	D	70)	A	B	C	D
12)	A	B	C	D	40)	A	B	C	D	71)	A	B	C	D
13)	A	B	C	D	41)	A	B	C	D	72)	A	B	C	D
14)	A	B	C	D	42)	A	B	C	D	73)	A	B	C	D
15)	A	B	C	D	43)	A	B	C	D	74)	A	B	C	D
16)	A	B	C	D	44)	A	B	C	D	75)	A	B	C	D
17)	A	B	C	D	45)	A	B	C	D	76)	A	B	C	D
18)	A	B	C	D	46)	A	B	C	D	77)	A	B	C	D
19)	A	B	C	D	47)	A	B	C	D	78)	A	B	C	D
20)	A	B	C	D	48)	A	B	C	D	79)	A	B	C	D
21)	A	B	C	D	49)	A	B	C	D	80)	A	B	C	D
22)	A	B	C	D	50)	A	B	C	D	81)	A	B	C	D
23)	A	B	C	D	51)	A	B	C	D	82)	A	B	C	D
24)	A	B	C	D	52)	A	B	C	D	83)	A	B	C	D
25)	A	B	C	D	53)	A	B	C	D	84)	A	B	C	D
26)	A	B	C	D	54)	A	B	C	D	85)	A	B	C	D
27)	A	B	C	D	55)	A	B	C	D	86)	A	B	C	D
28)	A	B	C	D	56)	A	B	C	D	87)	A	B	C	D
					57)	A	B	C	D	88)	A	B	C	D
					58)	A	B	C	D	89)	A	B	C	D
					59)	A	B	C	D	90)	A	B	C	D

91)	A	B	C	D	122)	A	B	C	D
92)	A	B	C	D	123)	A	B	C	D
93)	A	B	C	D	124)	A	B	C	D
94)	A	B	C	D	125)	A	B	C	D
95)	A	B	C	D	126)	A	B	C	D
96)	A	B	C	D	127)	A	B	C	D
97)	A	B	C	D	128)	A	B	C	D
98)	A	B	C	D	129)	A	B	C	D
99)	A	B	C	D	130)	A	B	C	D
100)	A	B	C	D	131)	A	B	C	D
101)	A	B	C	D	132)	A	B	C	D
102)	A	B	C	D	133)	A	B	C	D
103)	A	B	C	D	134)	A	B	C	D
104)	A	B	C	D	135)	A	B	C	D
105)	A	B	C	D	136)	A	B	C	D
106)	A	B	C	D	137)	A	B	C	D
107)	A	B	C	D	138)	A	B	C	D
108)	A	B	C	D	139)	A	B	C	D
109)	A	B	C	D	140)	A	B	C	D
110)	A	B	C	D	141)	A	B	C	D
111)	A	B	C	D	142)	A	B	C	D
112)	A	B	C	D	143)	A	B	C	D
113)	A	B	C	D	144)	A	B	C	D
114)	A	B	C	D	145)	A	B	C	D
115)	A	B	C	D	146)	A	B	C	D
116)	A	B	C	D	147)	A	B	C	D
117)	A	B	C	D	148)	A	B	C	D
118)	A	B	C	D	149)	A	B	C	D
119)	A	B	C	D	150)	A	B	C	D
120)	A	B	C	D					
121)	A	B	C	D					

Resources

Exam Preparation Products We Recommend

Medical Coding Exam Prep Course
http://medicalcodingpro.com/medical-coding-certification-prep-course/

Medical Coding Exam System
http://medicalcodingexamsystem.com

Faster Coder - Code Faster - Code Better
http://fastercoder.com

Other Resources

Elite Members Area – 7 day FREE trial!
http://medicalcodingpromembers.com

Medical Coding Pro – main website
http://medicalcodingpro.com

MEDICAL CODING PRO

Medical Coding Pro provides information about medical coding. We also help people in the medical coding community prepare for the medical coding certification exam.

Our mission is to help everyone we can pass the exam and gain their certification as quickly as possible.To do this we offer quality exam preparation tools such as Medical Coding Practice Exams, the Medical Coding Exam System, the Medical Coding Exam Strategy and the Medical Coding Pro Elite Members Area.

Visit us on the web at:

www.MedicalCodingPro.com

www.MedicalCodingProMembers.com

www.MedicalCodingExamSystem.com

www.MedicalCodingNews.org

Made in the USA
Columbia, SC
22 November 2019